Medieval Syphilis and Treponemal Disease

PAST IMPERFECT

See further
www.arc-humanities.org/our-series/pi

Medieval Syphilis and Treponemal Disease

Marylynn Salmon

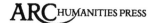

ARC HUMANITIES PRESS

British Library Cataloguing in Publication Data
A catalogue record for this book is available from the British Library

© 2022, Arc Humanities Press, Leeds

ISBN (print) 9781802700480
e-ISBN (PDF) 9781802700893
e-ISBN (EPUB) 9781802700909

www.arc-humanities.org
Printed and bound in the UK (by CPI Group [UK] Ltd), USA (by Bookmasters), and elsewhere using print-on-demand technology.

Contents

List of Illustrations

To Clive Holmes
in memorium

Preface and Acknowledgements

In April 2018 an interdisciplinary group of scholars in fields ranging from paleopathology and anthropological genetics to tropical medicine met in Santa Fe, New Mexico at the invitation of Gillian Crane-Kramer and Brenda J. Baker, and under the auspices of the School for Advanced Research. They wanted to discuss the state of research on the history and dissemination of treponematosis, including syphilis, a topic long debated in their community. This fruitful initial exchange led to two important events in March 2019: a symposium organized by Baker, "The Evolution of Syphilis: A New Approach," held at the 88th Annual Meeting of the American Association of Physical Anthropologists, and a workshop organized by Baker, Charlotte Roberts, Maciej Henneberg, and Ann Stodder on "Diagnosing Treponemal Disease" for the annual meeting of the Paleopathology Association. The result of all this effort was an article published in January 2020 in the *Yearbook of Physical Anthropology*, "Advancing the Understanding of Treponemal Disease in the Past and Present." Significantly for an academic publication, the authors listed their names alphabetically to signify their equal participation in this latest effort to understand the origin and spread of treponemal disease, among other topics. This short book is a response to a question posed in the article: Why have historians working with traditional manuscripts and works of art not found evidence of treponematosis before the sixteenth century?

An earlier version of this book was published as an article entitled "Evidence for the Presence of Treponemal Disease, Including Syphilis, in Late Medieval Europe" in issue 7.2 of the journal *The Medieval Globe* in 2021. I am grateful for the assistance of Carol Symes, Monica Green, and Arc Humanities Press in making it accessible here to a wider readership. For those wishing to explore this topic in greater depth, a full bibliography (unlike the Past Imperfect series's normal selective list of Further Reading) has been provided.

I also am indebted to Clive Holmes for commenting on the original version of this paper and encouraging me to publish it. Brenda J. Baker and Charlotte Roberts offered advice on compiling a list of cases of treponematosis, a delicate undertaking that they will undoubtedly say has not yet been successful. In addition, I appreciate the criticism of the anonymous referees, which encouraged me to solidify my evidence on a number of important points. Any remaining errors or weaknesses are, of course, my own. Finally, I am grateful to Carol Symes for recognizing the value of my work even though I am not trained as a medievalist, and for providing me with crucial translations and advice on word usage.

Introduction

Treponematosis, which takes several forms, including syphilis, is a painful and disfiguring disease that appears in a variety of guises depending on climate and social customs. For historians interested in the origins or dissemination of disease, treponematosis presents a particular challenge because it bears a close resemblance to several other illnesses. Even paleopathologists attest to the difficulty of identifying the disease in skeletal remains, although they have studied treponematosis intensively for decades to determine whether it arose in Europe before or after the voyages of Columbus—a culturally fraught investigative framework now rejected by many.

Despite significant controversy, the debate among paleopathologists over the presence of treponematosis in premodern Europe and in western Asia has finally been settled in the affirmative by the discovery of enough evidence from skeletal remains to satisfy even the staunchest of skeptics.[1]

---

[1] The best introduction to the theory that treponematosis was brought to Europe by the crew that sailed with Columbus is Harper et al., "The Origin and Antiquity of Syphilis Revisited" (2011). For the latest analysis of the pre-Columbian side of the debate see Baker et al., "Advancing the Understanding" (2020). Brenda J. Baker has been a leader in this long-running discussion, beginning with a highly influential article which she co-authored with George J. Armelagos comparing Old and New World skeletal

Yet it remains difficult to distinguish among the syndromes of the disease—bejel (*Treponema pallidum endemicum*), yaws (*Treponema pallidum pertenue*), and syphilis (*Treponema pallidum pallidum*)—that leave evidence in teeth and bones. (The fourth syndrome, pinta, or *Treponema pallidum carateum*, is a skin disease and therefore unrecoverable through paleopathology.) As the syndromes vary considerably in mortality rates and the level of human disgust they elicit, it is important to know which one is under discussion in any given case. Ancient DNA (aDNA) holds the answer, because just as only aDNA suffices to distinguish between treponematosis and other diseases that produce similar damage in the body, it alone can identify syndromes with absolute accuracy.[2] Progress on uncovering the historical extent of syndromes remains slow, however, because the spirochete responsible

---

evidence: "The Origin and Antiquity of Syphilis" (1988). They concluded that Columbus and his crew brought non-venereal treponematosis back to Spain, where it rapidly evolved into the venereal form of the disease due to climate and cultural factors. In now lending her support to the "pre-Columbian" hypothesis of the disease's presence in Europe because of new evidence in the field, Baker can be said to have started, and also to have ended, this stimulating scholarly debate.

2 Ancient DNA has proven to be particularly fruitful for the study of the origins and dissemination of the plague, and it is to be hoped that, in time, *Treponema pallidum* will be as well understood as *Yersinia pestis*. For an introduction to the possibilities of aDNA research on the plague, see the initial issue of *The Medieval Globe* (2014) edited by Monica Green, reprinted in *Pandemic Disease in the Medieval World* (2015). In December of 2020, Green published an important study on what she calls "The Four Black Deaths": the branches of *Yersinia pestis* that evolved at some point before the middle of the fourteenth century in an event colloquially termed the "Big Bang." She argues that the medieval pandemic emerged in central Eurasia by the thirteenth, not the fourteenth, century as a result of Mongol military campaigns, and that its fourteenth-century manifestation in Europe was a "spillover" event. Her work is heavily dependent on aDNA analysis derived from human and animal hosts.

for treponematosis, *treponema pallidum*, is rare in skeletal remains and fragile, making it notoriously difficult to recover and analyze. As a result, leaders in paleopathology have put out a call for more evidence of bejel, yaws, and syphilis from medieval documents and artworks to supplement their findings in teeth and bones. As observed by Brenda J. Baker and her co-authors, in their detailed and wide-ranging review of the literature published in 2020:

> Treponemal infection, particularly syphilis, has been a reviled and feared disease for centuries. This status marks syphilis as an issue for social commentary, not only through written documents, but also through artistic representations, and oral tales in many guises. It is time not only to reevaluate with a critical eye the written documents used to investigate the origins of treponemal infection, but also to include more fully the hitherto ignored but important sources of evidence—the pathographic and oral representations.[3]

Convincing evidence from traditional documentary and artistic sources will be difficult to obtain, however, as demonstrated by past failed efforts to prove that a particular disease was syphilis.[4] Certainly, descriptions of skin eruptions

---

3 Baker et al., "Advancing the Understanding" (2020), 18.

4 Holcomb, "The Antiquity of Syphilis" (1935), 297–303, citing a myriad of early medical writers although unfortunately without citations; Hudson, "Historical Approach to the Terminology of Syphilis" (1961), 545–50; Hackett, "Human Treponematoses" (1967). William Osler (1849–1919), the author of the first scientific medical textbook published in the United States, *The Principles and Practice of Medicine: Designed for the Use of Practitioners and Students of Medicine* (1892), famously told his students that syphilis was the only disease they needed to study thoroughly: "Know syphilis in all its manifestations and relations, and all other things clinical will be added unto you." This was often shortened to "Know syphilis, and know medicine." See his *Aequanimitas* (1910), 140. Osler's observation highlights why it has been so difficult to distinguish syphilis from other diseases in the historical record. Syphilis is also called "The Great Imitator."

and bone pain in medieval medical treatises sound like syphilis, but they could also be attributed to other diseases.[5]

This short book is a first attempt to examine traditional historical sources that offer evidence for the presence of treponematosis in medieval Europe. After considering the most relevant discoveries in clinical studies and paleopathology, I will turn to some remarkable documentary evidence for a single individual, the English king Edward IV (r. 1461–1470 and 1471–1483). I will argue that there is a clear reference to two forms of treponematosis, venereal (syphilis) and endemic (bejel), in a comment made by one of Edward's councillors about his death. A second contemporary observation provides supporting evidence, tracing a clear path forward toward establishing the existence of syphilis in late medieval England. Next, I will make a brief foray into the potentially rich but heretofore ambiguous evidence for the history of treponematosis in contemporary medical literature. I close with examples from medieval artworks that suggest how painters and illuminators might have portrayed symptoms of the disease. None of these contributions is intended to be definitive. The aim of this essay is to begin a conversation and encourage further research on the presence of treponemal disease in medieval Europe. While the most difficult challenge of establishing this fact has been completed at a preliminary level by paleopathologists, much detailed and innovative work will need to be done by scholars before we

---

5 For a clear and concise summary of the literature on this point see Baker and Armelagos, "The Origin and Antiquity of Syphilis" (1988), 705–7, 717. Overlooked in their study was an important overview of the historiography on the origins of treponematosis by Francisco Guerra, going back to the eighteenth century: "The Dispute over Syphilis" (1978). Guerra concluded (44, 55–57) that both endemic and venereal treponematosis existed in Europe before 1495, but not yaws, which he contended was introduced by the men who sailed with Columbus. In light of new scholarship, Guerra has retreated from this stance but has continued to maintain that "some form of treponematosis" existed in Europe before 1495: see his "European-American Exchange" (1993), 319.

can begin to evaluate the impact of treponematosis on the premodern world. For experts in the history of medicine, the history of sexuality, and art history, an exciting intellectual journey lies ahead. That it will be difficult is demonstrated by the evidence presented here, some of which may prove controversial.

Chapter 1

The Contributions of Clinicians and Paleopathologists

Medical understanding of the relationship between the different syndromes of treponematosis—bejel, yaws, and syphilis—was aided greatly by the work of a brilliant clinician working in the mid-twentieth century, Ellis Herndon Hudson (1890–1992). Among other investigations that have not been given their due by historians, he published an innovative study of endemic treponematosis titled *Non-Venereal Syphilis: A Sociological and Medical Study of Bejel* (1958). Hudson used the term "non-venereal" rather than "endemic" quite deliberately in his title, to impress upon readers his finding that bejel was devoid of the immoral connotations long associated with syphilis. He wanted them to understand that bejel, a disease of dry climates that thrived in the Middle East, was a childhood disease among the Bedouin, while syphilis was a disease of adults who lived in towns and cities. On the appearance of syphilis in urban areas, Hudson wrote, for example: "Venereal syphilis has no predilection for a particular climate, but it is found more in cities, where money is in freer circulation and amusements more organised; it is a companion of prostitution and other social behaviour problems."[1] He also cited a study of treponematosis in Bos-

---

1 Hudson, *Non-Venereal Syphilis* (1958), 3.

nia, concluding that "the prevalence of endemic syphilis was inversely proportional to the population."[2]

Hudson's seminal studies based on research in Syria and Iraq noted that habits of cleanliness, including keeping children fully clothed and indoors much of the time, were more common among urban dwellers, and he hypothesized that these conditions had led to the evolution of the venereal form of treponematosis in ancient cities.[3] To this crucial observation we should probably add a consideration of status, for elites led a very different lifestyle from the peasantry in stratified societies. Few elite children would be found scantily clad playing in the dirt of the stable yard or street, and generally not in the company of their social inferiors who might pass on a painful and unsightly disease through skin-to-skin contact or shared drinking vessels. The very fact that some people—whether urban dwellers, elites, or perhaps even Jews who observed strict rules on hygiene, clothing, and food consumption—did not become infected with endemic treponematosis in childhood made them susceptible to the venereal form of the disease as adults. Once the microorganism gained entry to the body through the genitals, the only way left open to it with all those protective clothes, it was much more serious than bejel and extremely difficult to treat before the advent of modern antibiotics.[4]

---

2 Hudson, *Non-Venereal Syphilis* (1958), 14. The study was by Ernest Grin and is discussed below.

3 Hudson, "Treponematosis and Man's Social Evolution" (1965), 894–95.

4 Ernest I. Grin concluded that the different outcomes of bejel and syphilis resulted from the significantly lower bacterial count found in endemic treponematosis: "Endemic Syphilis in Bosnia (1952)." As he writes, "The term 'endemic syphilis' subsequently became associated with non-venereal syphilis, usually acquired in childhood, in which repeated exposure to small numbers of treponemes over a period of time gives rise to the predominance of certain features not usually encountered in environments where venereal transmission makes a different age-group primarily susceptible." He cited (11) as

A lack of documentary evidence for the existence of syphilis in premodern Europe, combined with an explosion of sources attesting to the appearance of a "new" disease at the turn of the sixteenth century, led some historians to accept the opinions of contemporary medical writers that Columbus and his men had brought the disease from the New World to Spain. From there it spread rapidly.[5] In particular, the reliance of Charles VIII, king of France, on mercenary troops (some of them Spanish) at the time of his attack on Naples in the winter of 1495 had led, so the story went, to the dissemination of the highly contagious "Neapolitan disease" or "French pox" throughout Europe when those troops returned home to their own countries.[6]

Yet, as Hudson and other epidemiologists pointed out long ago, this explanation did not make sense in terms of what they then knew about the microorganism that causes treponematosis, including syphilis. It should have existed in Europe and neighbouring continents for centuries, if not millennia, and not been introduced all at once by people returning from a different hemisphere.[7] How, then, to reconcile the

conditions for endemic transmission "a low standard of education and poor economic and social conditions, with primitive sanitary and dwelling arrangements [...] these factors make for repeated exposure to treponemes, and the direct and indirect spread of disease is greatly facilitated." In venereal transmission (18), however, "A typical primary lesion usually develops after massive inoculation with treponemes—as, for instance, in a chancre of the nipple or on the genitalia." On superinfections of an already infected person Grin observes (25), "Little obstacle is opposed to repeated invasion of a sensitized human host by treponemes from the infected surroundings so long as the primitive living conditions of the population remain materially unchanged."

5 For an introduction to the literature, see Quétel, *History of Syphilis* (1990), 33–49.

6 On confusion about naming the new disease, see Quétel, *History of Syphilis* (1990), 13–16.

7 Hudson, "Historical Approach to the Terminology of Syphilis" (1961), 561.

contradiction between an emerging scientific understanding and gaps in the historical record? An obvious solution to the problem came from the field of paleopathology, with its objective evidence extracted from skeletal remains to supplement written sources such as chronicle accounts and medical treatises. If skeletons with deformities symptomatic of treponematosis could be discovered and analyzed, they would prove that the disease had existed in medieval or even ancient Europe and so contribute to the validation or dismissal of the Columbian hypothesis.

Despite the existence of thousands of bones in museum collections and many hundreds of skeletons excavated from historic burial sites, uncovering examples of treponemal disease in the Old World has turned out to be a surprisingly difficult endeavour. One important reason is treponemal lesions' lack of specificity. The same kinds of bone lesions result from a number of different diseases, making it difficult, and in most cases impossible, to differentiate among them. At the same time, the scarring that is pathognomonic of treponematosis—advanced decay, *caries sicca* of the skull, and gummatous lesions on tubular bones—have low sensitivity, meaning that the number of cases in any population is going to be small.[8] Moreover, while evidence from bones will survive if treponematosis is present at the time of death, most cases produce no lesions at all. Estimates vary, but paleopathologists believe that bone lesions severe enough to result in permanent damage appear in at most about 20 percent of cases.[9] Thus, in a study of 219 adult and 53 child and adolescent skeletons excavated in Metaponto in southern Italy (580–250

---

8 Baker et al., "Advancing the Understanding" (2020), 19.

9 Harper et al., "The Origin and Antiquity of Syphilis Revisited" (2011), 101. See also Walker et al., "Evidence of Skeletal Treponematosis" (2015), 91: the authors give a figure of 10–12 percent for venereal treponematosis, the most virulent form of the disease. The figure is even smaller when venereal treponematosis is excluded. Baker and Armelagos note, of New World evidence, that "It must be reiterated that bone lesions are expected in only 1–5 percent of individuals

BCE), only 45 of the total 272 show bone abnormalities possibly indicative of treponemal disease.[10] And out of 5,387 skeletons excavated in the cemetery at St. Mary Spital (the priory of St. Mary without Bishopsgate) in London (1120–1539 CE), only twenty-five show signs of infection.[11] Simon Mays and colleagues similarly note that examples of treponemal infection are rare even in British collections from the eighteenth and nineteenth centuries, "despite the fact that by that time syphilis was firmly established, particularly in urban populations."[12]

The evidence from surviving dental tissue has turned out to be less ambiguous. It has long been recognized that certain deformities, specifically Hutchinson's notched incisors and Moon's domed or mulberry shaped molars, are pathognomonic of treponemal disease. (The names refer to the pathologists, Jonathan Hutchinson and Henry Moon, who first categorized them in the nineteenth century.) In addition, common variations of these abnormalities are also now regarded as specific to the disease.[13] As with bones, not all skeletons demonstrate these dental abnormalities; but estimates as high as forty-five, sixty, or even sixty-five percent indicate there are many more examples yet to

---

in skeletal series from areas in which yaws or endemic syphilis occurred": "The Origin and Antiquity of Syphilis" (1988), 719.

10 Henneberg and Henneberg, "Treponematosis in an Ancient Greek Colony" (1994), 92. They also found two cases of dental abnormalities, making their total forty-seven cases of treponematosis.

11 Walker et al., "Evidence of Skeletal Treponematosis" (2015), 90.

12 On the scarcity of evidence they observe: "It was present in only 2 skeletons of 968 from 18th–19th century Christ Church Spitalfields, London, and there is one example each from collections of similar date excavated from Red Cross Way, London (N=148 skeletons) and Kingston-upon-Thames, near London (N=360)." See Mays, Crane-Kramer, and Bayliss, "Two Probable Cases of Treponemal Disease" (2003), 140.

13 Ioannou, Henneberg, and Henneberg, "Presence of Dental Signs" (2018), 192–93.

discover.[14] And although variations in the presentation of treponematosis have resulted in considerable debate among scholars in the past, consensus is growing on what constitutes a valid diagnosis, to the extent that scholars are now able to differentiate between cases that were and were not treated with mercury.[15] Still, the small number of confirmed cases has been frustrating.

Complicating the ability of paleopathologists to diagnose treponematosis is the virtual impossibility of distinguishing among bejel, yaws, and syphilis in the analysis of dental tissue. In all three syndromes, the teeth can be affected in similar ways because, while transplacental transmission is rare in bejel and yaws due to the latent nature of the disease in most women of childbearing age, it can occur.[16] As Baker and her co-authors have observed, however, "Despite the demonstrated occurrence of congenital transmission in yaws and bejel, CS [congenital syphilis] is typically conceived as a proxy for the presence of sexually acquired syphilis in a mother."[17] They argue that such proxy designations should no longer be used as proof of the existence of syphilis in a particular case because even Hutchinson's incisors, once considered the gold standard for a diagnosis of the disease, are now known to be reliable only for congenital treponematosis generally, not individual syndromes.[18] Using evidence from the teeth alone to

---

14 The forty-five percent estimate for Hutchinson's incisors comes from Putoken, "Dental Changes" (1962). The sixty percent estimate comes from Hillson, *Dental Anthropology* (1996), 171–72. The sixty-five percent estimate comes from Goens, Janniger, and De Wolf, "Dermatologic and Systemic Manifestations" (1994), 1013–21.

15 Ioannou et al., "Diagnosing Congenital Syphilis" (2016), 617. See also Ioannou, Henneberg, and Henneberg, "Presence of Dental Signs" (2018), 192–200.

16 Akwari, "Is Bejel Syphilis?" (1949), especially 118; Grin, "Endemic Syphilis in Bosnia" (1952), especially 31–33, 70; Román and Román, "Occurrence" (1986), especially 764–65.

17 Baker et al. "Advancing the Understanding" (2020), 19.

18 Of bejel among the Bedouin in Iraq, Akwari reports: "Among

distinguish among bejel, yaws, and syphilis is just not possible. That said, because yaws is a subtropical disease, it is undoubtedly rare, although not nonexistent, in northern climates.[19]

Neither does surviving bone evidence usually offer much assistance in distinguishing among treponemal syndromes. Tibial bowing is indicative of treponematosis contracted during childhood because it is common in both bejel and yaws, but it may also appear in cases of congenital syphilis, or even in cases of syphilis contracted in adulthood when it presents as pseudo-bowing with newly created anterior surface bone deposited on top of older tissue. Bone striations and pitting similarly occur in all three syndromes. The exception to this generalization is cranial involvement, which is rare in cases of both bejel and yaws. In particular, calvarial (top of the skull) damage is considered highly diagnostic for syphilis.[20] Finally, extensive destruction of both long bones and those of the cranium in the same specimen occurs much more often in venereal cases. Given this reality, Don Walker and his co-authors have called for recognition of the sheer amount of bone destruction in some skeletons as pathognomonic of venereal treponematosis.[21]

The difficult question of whether bone specimens hold evidence of treponematosis rather than some other dis-

---

218 persons of one tribe examined without selection in the Ramadi district, we found five with typical Hutchinson's teeth and thirty-one with saddle noses. Seventy-three of the 218 were children between the ages of 1 and 15 years. Most of the saddle noses were observed in the latter group." See Akwari, "Is Bejel Syphilis?" (1949), 118.

19 Giffin et al. "A Treponemal Genome" (2020).

20 The extensive work of Cecil J. Hackett in museum collections is considered authoritative on this question. On *caries sicca*, see his *Diagnostic Criteria of Syphilis* (1976), 30–49; on calvarial destruction, 49–63; on destruction of the facial bones, 63–66; on long bones, 76–97. See also Ortner, *Identification of Pathological Conditions* (2003), 280; and Steinbock, *Paleopathological Diagnosis* (1976), 139, 143.

21 Walker et al., "Evidence of Skeletal Treponematosis" (2015), 91, 93–94, 97.

ease, such as tuberculosis or bacterial osteomyelitis, can be answered by DNA and aDNA evidence. The genetic sequence of the spirochete responsible for treponematosis was deciphered in 1998 and success in analyzing a 200-year-old example extracted from bones came the next year.[22] Further progress in isolating specimens from bone samples has been painfully slow, however, due largely to the fragile nature of the organism and its rarity in surviving bones and teeth.[23] Then, in 2012, Rafael Montiel and his co-authors decided to focus on skeletons demonstrative of congenital syphilis on the assumption that those bones would hold higher bacterial loads than were present in adolescent or adult skeletons. Their hypothesis was correct, and they were successful in amplifying two *Treponema pallidum* DNA sequences, proving that the congenital variant of treponematosis is the key to advancing future work in the field. But again, because the evidence used in this study is identical in cases of bejel, yaws, and syphilis—and because the bones were dated to the sixteenth and seventeenth centuries—this innovative work was not useful in addressing the debate on the origin of syphilis in premodern Europe or its neighbouring continents.[24]

Recent progress in studying congenital syphilis continues to yield exciting results, due to technological innovations that include short DNA fragment extraction, targeted DNA enrichment, and "next-generation" whole genome sequencing.[25] In 2018, using this advanced technology, Verena J. Schuen-

---

22 Fraser et al., "Complete Genome Sequence" (1998); Kolman et al., "Identification of *Treponema Pallidum* Subspecies *Pallidum*" (1999).

23 A number of studies published shortly after Kolman et al. concluded that it was not possible to extract treponemal DNA from human bones: including Bouwman and Brown, "The Limits of Biomolecular Palaeopathology" (2005); and Von Hunnius et al., "Digging Deeper" (2007).

24 Montiel et al., "Neonate Human Remains" (2012).

25 Baker et al., "Advancing the Understanding" (2020), 9–10, citing Stone and Ozga, "Ancient DNA in the Study of Ancient Disease" (2019).

emann and colleagues successfully recovered and reconstructed *Treponema pallidum* genomes from the skeletons of two infants and a neonate interred in the historic cemetery of the Convent of Santa Isabel in Mexico City, in operation from 1681 to 1861. Two are believed to have had congenital syphilis and one congenital yaws.[26]

A breakthrough example from early modern Europe can be found in the work of Karen Giffin and her co-authors, who recently sequenced a genome of *Treponema pallidum* subspecies *pertenue*, the causal agent of yaws, from a Lithuanian tooth radiocarbon-dated to 1447–1616 (95 percent probability).[27] The ability to sequence the entire genome is especially important for distinguishing among syndromes of treponematosis because they are 99.8 percent genetically identical. In this case, whole genome sequencing has resulted in two startling discoveries: that the subtropical syndrome yaws existed in northern Europe at the turn of the sixteenth century, and that yaws in its modern form is a relatively young disease that emerged only in the twelfth to fourteenth centuries. As a result of their success, Giffin and colleagues are highly optimistic about the future of a DNA analysis in paleopathology, observing that concern about the inaccessibility of evidence for treponemal diseases in archaeological material has discouraged researchers for too long. They conclude, "As the roster of archaeological samples showing molecular preservation of these diseases increases, and their detection is further enhanced by analytical advances, the resolution of enigmas related to the origins of the full treponemal cluster, inclusive of its other members syphilis, bejel, and pinta, are within reach."[28]

In October 2020 Kerttu Majander and colleagues published research revealing that as early as the fifteenth to

---

26 Schuenemann et al., "Historic *Treponema Pallidum* Genomes" (2018).

27 Giffin et al. "A Treponemal Genome" (2020), 6.

28 Giffin et al. "A Treponemal Genome" (2020), 11.

eighteenth centuries *Treponema pallidum* existed as syphilis and yaws in Finland, syphilis in Estonia, and a previously unknown basal strain in the Netherlands. Although precise dating is not yet possible, the presence of several different kinds of treponematosis at the beginning of the early modern period argues against its recent introduction from elsewhere. Therefore, they argue, treponematosis—including syphilis—almost certainly existed in medieval Europe.[29]

Despite significant progress in identifying treponemal disease in European skeletal remains, the number of cases from the medieval period remains small, primarily due to the difficulty of achieving scholarly consensus. To date, six examples of congenital treponematosis based on evidence from teeth and fifteen cases of acquired treponematosis based on evidence from bones are widely accepted. In four of the twenty-one cases the evidence may also indicate syphilis. Because this literature is not well known to historians, a summary is included here in chronological order. The cases most indicative of syphilis are starred, but readers should keep in mind that even these diagnoses are not regarded as definitive. The dating of some skeletal remains to the pre-Columbian period also continues to spark debate.

1–2. The most ancient skeletal examples of treponematosis in Europe come from southern Italy circa 580–225 BCE. Two burials, both of adolescents, yield dental evidence of congenital treponematosis, specifically Hutchinson's incisors and Moon's molars. Such dentition is considered necessary for an accurate diagnosis as no other disease produces these effects, but it cannot distinguish between the endemic and venereal forms of the disease.[30]

*3. A burial of a young male in the Apple Down cemetery near Up Marden, West Sussex in the United Kingdom, radio-

---

29 See their "Ancient Bacterial Genomes" (2020), 3796.

30 Henneberg and Henneberg, "Treponematosis in an ancient Greek colony (1994)," 92–98. For additional discussion of these cases see Ioannou, Henneberg, and Henneberg, "Presence of Dental Signs of Congenital Syphilis (2018)," 192–200.

carbon-dated to the sixth century CE, reveals evidence of treponematosis in *caries sicca* of the skull and gummatous lesions of the long bones. *Caries sicca*, like Hutchinson's incisors, is considered pathognomonic of acquired treponematosis, but the characteristic pits and cavitation may be produced by either the endemic or venereal forms of the disease. That said, involvement of the skull in bejel and yaws is regarded as rare. Significantly, evidence of the deceased's high social status as seen in the range of burial goods found in the grave also points to venereal rather than endemic treponematosis. As the authors observe of their diagnosis, "The factors taken into account in this decision, made on the basis of probabilities, include the geographical pathogen range, the apparent low prevalence of the disease at this large cemetery, the high social status of the individual, the presence of social upheaval at the time, and the early age of death of the individual. These factors should be considered in their totality."[31]

4. The dentition of a two to three-year-old child with multiple examples of Hutchinson's incisors and Moon's molars from Hamage, France has been by dated by the authors to the seventh to eighth century CE, although they include no information about their methods.[32]

5. The skeleton of a child aged seven to nine years with Hutchinson's incisors and Moon's molars was exhumed from a cemetery near Trolla's Chapel in Kintradwell, Scotland. It has been radiocarbon dated to 1040-1280 CE. Poignantly, the child was buried with little treasures—a cow's tooth and a red pebble.[33]

*6. A burial of a teenager in thirteenth-century Nicaea in western Anatolia holds pathological evidence of trepo-

---

[31] Cole and Waldron, "Apple Down 152: A Putative Case of Syphilis (2011)," 72–79. See also their "Letter to the Editor: Syphilis Revisited (2012)," 149–50; and for the quotation, Cole and Waldron, "Letter to the Editor: Pre-Colombian Date Confirmed (2014)," 489.

[32] Blondiaux, "La Paléopathologie des tréponématoses" (2008), 453–62.

[33] Lelong and Roberts, "St. Trolla's Chapel" (2003), 147–63 at 159.

nematosis in the dentition, including a Hutchinson's incisor and a Moon's molar. Bone evidence includes saber tibia, dactylitis, and gummatous and non-gummatous lesions "on almost every post-cranial bone." Involvement of both teeth and bones in the same individual, and especially the large number of bones affected, are regarded as strong evidence, albeit not proof, of syphilis. The dating of this case caused debate because radiocarbon dating was not possible. In the end the quality of traditional archaeological evidence commonly employed for dating, including coins found in situ, was determined to be definitive.[34]

7. In the Church of Saint Idzi in Wrocław, Poland the exhumation of a probable fourteenth-century burial revealed a skeleton with evidence of treponematosis. Extensive *caries sicca* of the skull is accompanied by infectious damage to one femur and one tibia. The authors did not include information on how they arrived at the dating of the skeleton beyond associating it with the age of the church.[35]

*8–9. The medieval cemetery of St. Mary Spital in London contains seven burials of individuals with symptoms of treponematosis radiocarbon dated to before 1400. Two of these have been the focus of detailed analysis aimed at demonstrating the existence of syphilis in skeletal remains. Both specimens have numerous postcranial gummatous and non-gummatous lesions and extensive deposits of periosteal new bone. One also has a surviving skull with *caries sicca*, a pairing viewed by many paleopathologists as crucial for indicating the disease. As the authors observe, "Yaws, endemic syphilis [bejel], and venereal syphilis [syphilis] can all produce similar bone changes and are difficult to distinguish.

---

34 Erdal, "A Pre-Columbian Case of Congenital Syphilis from Anatolia (2006)," 16–33 at 16. See also Ioannou, Henneberg, and Henneberg, "Presence of Dental Signs of Congenital Syphilis (2018)," 195–96, and Ioannou et al., "Diagnosing Congenital Syphilis (2016)," 626.

35 Gładykowska-Rzeczycka et al., "Treponematosis in a 14th-Century Skeleton" (2003), 187–93.

Differences in skeletal involvement between the diseases are to a certain extent quantitative; with the cranial vault rarely involved in endemic syphilis and yaws." They conclude that the evidence points to syphilis in this one case largely because of calvarial involvement combined with extensive postcranial bone destruction.[36]

10. A medieval cemetery in St. Pölten, Austria contains the remains of a child aged approximately six years buried between 1390 and 1440 according to radiocarbon dating. The dentition displays Hutchinson's incisors and Moon's molars consistent with congenital treponematosis.[37]

*11, 12–16. St. Margaret's cemetery in Norwich, UK received burials between 1254 and 1468, when it was closed. The land subsequently reverted to agricultural uses. Archaeological dating is therefore highly dependable for this cemetery. Excavations revealed six burials with evidence of treponematosis, one with both *caries sicca* and changes to "most of the post-cranial skeleton." As we have seen, this combination is highly suggestive of syphilis. Two other skeletons with *caries sicca* and postcranial bone damage, two with extensive bilateral long bone damage (one radiocarbon dated to the medieval period), and one with *caries sicca* but without significant postcranial bone damage, comprise the group.[38]

17. A young adult female buried in the cemetery of the Dominican Friary of Blackfriars in Gloucester, UK has been dated from 1239 to the mid-fifteenth century by traditional archaeological methods. This skeleton holds widespread evidence of treponematosis ranging from *caries sicca* and nasopalatine destruction on the skull (saddle nose, a distinctive facial deformity of treponematosis) to numerous lesions on the long bones, ribs, clavicles, scapulae, and sternum. This

---

36 Walker et al., "Evidence of Skeletal Treponematosis (2015)," 90–101 at 91.

37 Gaul et al., "A Probable Case of Congenital Syphilis (2015)," 451–72.

38 Stirland, *Criminals and Paupers*, 28–35 at 28. See also her earlier "Evidence for Pre-Columbian Treponematosis" (1994), 114–15.

combination makes it a good candidate for a diagnosis of syphilis, but the author believes that joint destruction of the kind found in this skeleton is more typical of yaws.[39]

18–19. Research on historic cemeteries in Denmark produced two pre-Columbian burials of individuals with treponemal disease. One of these, radiocarbon dated to the mid-fifteenth century, shows *caries sicca* of the skull as well as multiple lesions on three long bones. The other, from a cemetery securely dated by traditional archaeological methods to the period 1100 to 1350, has damage only to the skull. In this case the combination of serpiginous lesions on the frontal bone and remodeling of the nasal aperture and inferior nasal conchae is significant because it points to saddle nose.[40]

20–21. In a rural cemetery in Rivenhall, Essex, the skeletal remains of a female aged 25 to 50 years exhibit signs of treponemal disease in eleven long bones, accompanied by erosive joint lesions. According to radiocarbon dating, the bones are pre-Columbian with 99 percent certainty. In nearby Ipswich another burial of a female aged about fifty shows similar pathological changes in ten long bones. This skeleton retains the skull, which shows erosions on the outer table accompanied by sclerotic thickening also indicative of treponematosis. Radiocarbon dating to before 1493 is only 73 percent certain in this case, but the authors note that the age of the deceased, combined with the necessity for treponematosis to be present in the body for decades before the bones can be affected to this degree, mean the probability is much higher that the burial occurred before the end of the fifteenth century. Significantly, this woman was buried in the nave of the Blackfriars church, indicating that she was a person of high status. In neither case can the exact nature of the infection—endemic or venereal—be determined, but the authors

39 Roberts, "Treponematosis in Gloucester, England" (1994), 101–8. On yaws, see p. 105. On the dating of this case, see also Harper, "The Origin and Antiquity of Syphilis Revisited" (2011), 111.

40 Schwarz, Skytte, and Rasmussen, "Treponemal Infection in Denmark?" (2013), 19.

note that the women probably suffered from the same disease because their lesions were similar.[41]

This survey of the literature in paleopathology demonstrates that treponematosis existed in Europe and western Asia well before contact with the Western Hemisphere, perhaps—given the work of Maciej and Renata J. Henneberg (1994)—even before the establishment of the Roman Empire. But the evidence remains sparse and localized, while specific syndromes are debatable. For this reason, Baker and her co-authors have called for a more systematic approach to analyzing and categorizing tissue samples with field-wide inclusion of the same information on location, dating, and demographic profiles of evidence, in order to improve analysis of such key issues as environmental conditions (climate, altitude) and variation across time or cultures (clothing, drinking vessels). Of particular importance to historians, they have noted the key role that documentary and artistic evidence may play in advancing our understanding not only of the origin, but also the lived experience, of treponemal disease. Their call for more evidence from traditional sources gives my examination of the admittedly sparse material on the death of Edward IV greater importance than it might otherwise hold, for it allows me to compare symptoms of endemic and venereal treponematosis in elites and commoners.

---

41 Mays, Crane-Kramer, and Bayliss, "Two Probable Cases of Treponemal Disease (2003)," 133–43.

Chapter 2

Deciphering Two Opaque Sources on the Death of King Edward IV of England

The once-warlike King Edward IV of England died in his bed on April 9, 1483, aged only forty. The royal council gave no official explanation for his death. This naturally led to confusion, and contemporary commentators speculated about the causes. They reported variously that he died of apoplexy, melancholy, or fevers.[1] Modern historians remain perplexed. Charles Ross, Edward IV's most scholarly biographer, concludes that it is impossible to know what killed the king, although his notorious self-indulgence was surely a factor.[2] In pointing to the king's gluttony, Ross was following his predecessor, the eminent early twentieth-century historian Cora Scofield, who believed it likely that Edward had died from a stroke, or perhaps acute indigestion, citing the contemporary French chroniclers Thomas Basin (1412–1491) and Jean de Roye (ca. 1425–ca. 1490) as her authorities.[3] In making

---

1 Ross provides a summary of the evidence in his *Edward IV*, 414–16.

2 Ross, *Edward IV*, 415.

3 Basin, *Histoire des règnes*, 3:133–34. "However, another none-too-small misfortune also happened for the kingdom of the English at this time from the quite sudden and untimely death of its king Edward. For when on the holy day of Venus [April 1], in the year 1483 (by the custom of the Roman Curia), the same king, for the sake of devotion and prayer, had purified many churches and sacred places, afterwards both restoring his tired body and

her conjecture, Scofield emphasized the king's unhealthy lifestyle. As she observed, "Had Death delayed his work three
weeks longer, Edward would have been forty-one years old.
It was an early age for a man to die, even then when the
average life span was considerably shorter than it is today;
but for libertinism and high living, to both of which, there is
no doubt, Edward was much given, even the strongest consti-
tution must sooner or later pay the price."[4]

In spite of the mystery surrounding the king's death, Ross
and Scofield could point quite confidently to the ill effects
of this self-indulgence because contemporaries did not hold
back in their criticism of the king. A chronicler of Crowland (or
Croyland) Abbey in Lincolnshire, for example, describes him
as "a gross man [...] addicted to conviviality, vanity, drunken-
ness, extravagance, and passion." At another place, he writes
that the king "indulged too intemperately his own passions

---

refilling himself with fruits and vegetables, abstaining from wine,
with a disease having been contracted, within eight days he ended
his unstable rule together with his life." The Latin reads: "Contigit
autem et regno Anglorum aliud non parvum infortunium, ea
tempestate, de subita satis et immatura regis sui morte Edoardi.
Nam cum die veneris sanctae, anno MCCCCLXXXIII more romanae
curiae, idem rex, devotionis et orationis causa, plures ecclesias
et loca sacra perlustrasset, postmodum quoque reficiens lassum
corpus, et fructibus atque oleribus vino abstinens replesset se,
contracto morbo, infra dies octo instabile regnum simul cum vita
finivit." I would like to thank Aaron Hershkowitz for providing the
translation. De Roye reports that he had heard the story this way
(Journal, 2:130): "In the month of April, King Edward of England
died in the kingdom of an apoplexy which affected him. Others
say that he was poisoned while drinking the good wine from the
Creu de Challuau that the king had given him, from which he
drank in such abundance that he died." The French reads, "Oudit
mois d'avril, le roy Edouart d'Angleterre mourut oudit royaulme
d'une apoplexie qui le print. Autres disent qu'il fut empoisonné en
buvant du bon vin du creu de Challuau que le roy luy avoit donné,
duquel il but en si grande habondance qu'il en morut."

4 Scofield, *Life and Reign*, 2:366. Philippe de Commines also says
that Edward died of apoplexy: *Memoirs*, 2:413.

and desire for luxury."[5] Domenico Mancini, an Italian visitor to London at the time of, or shortly after, Edward's death, adds detail to this picture, reporting that "In food and drink he was most immoderate: it was his habit, so I have learned, to take an emetic for the delight of gorging his stomach once more. For this reason, and for the ease, which was especially dear to him after the recovery of his crown, he had grown fat in the loins."[6]

In addition to overeating and drinking, the king was known for indulging his sexual appetites in an extravagant manner. Those who noted Edward's reputation for lechery included John Hardyng, a contemporary who described the young king as "a man that loved both to see and feele a fayre woman."[7] Mancini learned from conversations with courtiers that Edward was "licentious in the extreme.[...] He pursued with no discrimination the married and the unmarried, the noble and lowly: however, he took none by force."[8] Similar opinions

---

5 *The Crowland Chronicle Continuations*, trans. Pronay and Cox, 153, 151. The Latin reads, "homine tam corpulento tantis solidalitiis, vanitatibus, crapulis, luxui et cupiditatibus" and "licet diebus suis cupiditatibus et luxui nimis intemperanter indulsisse creditur."

6 Mancini, *De occupatione*, ed. and trans. as *Usurpation* by Armstrong, 67. The Latin reads: "Cibi et potus fuit intemperantissimus. Vomitum provocare solitum accepi, ut voluptate edendi iterum stomachum referciret. Propter hoc et ocium, quod post confirmatum regnum valde ei amicum fuit, pinguis ad abdomen devenerat." Mancini was almost certainly employed by the prominent Neapolitan physician and astrologer, Angelo Cato, archbishop of Vienne, for whom he wrote his account of the English court in 1483. Cato was at this period a counsellor and physician of Louis XI of France, so he was probably collecting information for the king. Mancini did not speak English and was therefore dependent on informants who could speak to him in Italian or Latin. There would have been many such men at court.

7 *Chronicle of John Hardyng*, ed. Ellis, 439n1.

8 Mancini, *Usurpation*, ed. and trans. Armstrong, 67. "Libidinis ut fuit intemperantissimus, ita in multas mulieres postquam eis potitus fuerat, fertur fuisse contumeliosus. [...] Nuptas et innuptas: matronas atque humiles nullo discrimine egit, nullam tamen vi rapuit."

circulating on the Continent led the French diplomat Philippe de Commines (1447–1511) to ascribe Edward's temporary loss of his throne in 1470–1471 to his love of pleasure.[9] Indeed, the king's sexual reputation was so entrenched that it lasted into the reign of his grandson Henry VIII, whose lord chancellor Thomas More wrote that Edward was "greatly given to fleshly wantonness."[10] Yet indulging at table and in bed do not usually kill men as young as Edward, which may be why some people believed the king had been poisoned: so at least reported Polydore Vergil (ca. 1470–1555), historian to Henry VII (r. 1485–1509).[11] It therefore seems worth looking more closely at contemporary accounts of Edward's death to try to unravel the mystery. When we do, opaque comments by the Crowland chronicler and Mancini become particularly useful.

Nicholas Pronay and John Cox, editors of the anonymous continuations of the *Crowland Chronicle*, believe that the author was probably a member of the king's council because he was familiar with the court and its workings.[12] Never-

---

9 de Commines, *Memoirs*, 1:217.

10 More, *History of King Richard III*, ed. Logan, 5.

11 Vergil, *Three Books*, ed. Ellis, 172. The "poison" may have been mercury, a point discussed further below.

12 Pronay and Cox, "The Riddle of Authorship" in their edition of *The Crowland Chronicle Continuations*, 78–95. They propose Bishop John Russell as the author, an attribution that remains unproved. Michael Hicks proposes Master Richard Langport, clerk of the king's council: see his "The Second Anonymous Continuation," 362–69. Hicks notes that others who have been proposed are John Gunthorpe, dean of Wells, royal chaplain, and diplomat; Richard Lavender, archdeacon of Leicester and doctor of canon law; Henry Sharp, doctor of civil law, royal clerk, and diplomat; Piers Curteys, keeper first of the palace at Westminster and then of the Great Wardrobe. Because of their positions, these men might well have been as knowledgeable as Russell about the cause of Edward's death. In response to Hicks, Alison Hanham argues that it was not an insider at court who penned this part of the chronicle, but a member of the Crowland community, probably the prior Richard Cambridge. His knowledge of the court and diplomacy

theless, rather than saying outright what killed Edward—although he was presumably in a position to know—the chronicler wrote cryptically that "while the king himself was not old, and not potentially afflicted anywhere with a definitely known kind of disease, of which the cure in a person of lesser status would not be considered easy, he fell into his bed around Eastertide and on the 9th day of April gave up his spirit."[13] This opinion seems to contradict the authorities Scofield and Ross followed in making their assessments, for practitioners of medicine in the fifteenth century recognized a stroke when they saw one. Two aspects of the chronicler's comment then become important for understanding what did kill the king: his belief that the disease was unknown, and that it was harder to cure in an elite person than in one of lower status.

The claim that Edward died of an unknown illness—that is, one not discussed in the contemporary medical literature—is an important key to understanding its nature because it suggests treponematosis. Only following the French invasion of Italy by Charles VIII, and the dissemination of reports that his mercenary troops were infected with a horrific venereal disease, did physicians begin to write about the symptoms and treatment of what we call syphilis. They often commented, moreover, that it was a previously unknown disease. But now

---

during the reign of Edward IV would have come from insiders who reported events to him: see Hanham, "Mysterious Affair," 6, 11.

13 *The Crowland Chronicle Continuations*, trans. Pronay and Cox, 151: this translation is by Carol Symes. The Latin reads: "cum rex ille neque senior, neque quovis intellect certo genere morbi cujus cura in minori persona facilis non videretur affectus esset, decidit in lectum circiter festum Paschae as nono die Aprilus Creatori sui spiritum reddidit apud palatium suum Westmonasterii, anno Domini millesimo quadringentesimo octagesimo tertio et anno regni sui vicesimo tertio." The chronicler's prose is sometimes acknowledged to be opaque. As observed by Hicks, his Latin "was laconic, allusive and ambiguous, perhaps deliberately, so that some readings are contested and probably insoluble": "The Second Anonymous Continuation," 352.

that we have physical evidence for the existence of treponematosis in medieval Europe, this seems very strange. How could a distinctive disease that was to reach epidemic proportions at the turn of the sixteenth century be unrecognized and denied a name only a short time earlier?

The most likely explanation is that syphilis, and bejel as well, were not "unknown" but rather confused with other diseases having similar symptoms, including leprosy, mentagra, tzara'ath, elephantiasis, scabies, and boa or bova. Over the centuries, the names and descriptions of these diseases evolved and shifted depending on local exposure and new ideas about how they were related. As Hudson observes of boa, in his study of medical terminology, "Thus it is possible to link boa the 'snake disease' with 'serpedo' of Isidore (7th C.) (which he in turn related to 'leprosy'), with the 'serpentine leprosy' of Albucasis (10th C.), and with the Serpentine Disease of [Ruy Díaz] de Isla (1539) that he said was called bubas."[14] The variety of symptoms of treponematosis, the different ages at which the disease appears, and its widely divergent outcomes, would have added greatly to the confusion of medical practitioners, as indeed they did right into the middle of the twentieth century.

One disease that was almost certainly confused with treponematosis in both the ancient and medieval worlds is Hansen's Disease (leprosy), sometimes called venereal leprosy.[15] Thus, symptoms of treponematosis were often assigned to "leprosy" erroneously. Both syphilis and bejel are highly contagious; however, Hansen's Disease is difficult to trans-

---

14 See Hudson, "Historical Approach to the Terminology of Syphilis" (1961), 67.

15 As Holcomb observes, "Among those who wrote of venereal leprosy are the Spanish surgeon Alzaharavius, the Italian surgeon Theodoric [Borgognoni], the Parisian professor Batholomeus Angelicus, the Scottish professor at Montpelier, Bernard Gordon, the two Englishmen Gilbert Anglicus, and John Gaddesden, and the Portuguese Velascus of Tarentum. There are many others." See his "The Antiquity of Syphilis" (1935), 297.

mit because ninety-five percent of people are immune to the bacteria, *Mycobacterium leprae*, that causes it.[16] Yet leprosy was wrongly believed to be so contagious that, for centuries, sufferers were required to live separately from their communities, denied entrance even to churches. Moreover, syphilis is readily transmitted through sexual intercourse, whereas Hansen's Disease is not, despite the fact that many medieval physicians believed leprosy could be caught by having sexual relations with someone infected with the disease. Claims that leprosy was inheritable can also be discredited: it is actually impossible, because *Mycobacterium leprae* cannot cross the placenta during pregnancy—although *Treponema pallidum* can.[17] Nor can leprosy be treated with mercury as syphilis can, although during the Middle Ages sufferers diagnosed with leprosy were often given mercury both internally

---

[16] This figure comes from the Centers for Disease Control and Prevention: https://www.cdc.gov/leprosy/transmission/index.html (retrieved August 7, 2021).

[17] Holcomb, "The Antiquity of Syphilis" (1935), 298–99. Bartholomaeus Anglicus (before 1203–1272) wrote a description of leprosy in his *De proprietatibus rerum* that fits syphilis much better, here in the translation of Stephen Batman or Bateman (1582), *Batman vppon Bartholome his Booke De Proprietatibus Rerum*, chap. 65: "Lepra commeth of diuerse causes besides the foresayde humours, as of dwelling and inhabiting and kéeping-companye, and oft talking with leprous men. For the euill is contagious, & infecteth other men. Also it commeth of fleshlye lyking, by a woman soone after that a leprous man hath laye by her. Also it commeth of Father and mother: and so this contagion passeth into the childe as it were by lawe of heritage. And sometime it falleth when a childe is conceyued in menstruall time: And also when a childe is fedde with corrupt milke of a leprous Nurse." According to Holcomb, Theodoric Burgognoni was particularly observant about modes of transmission, noting that if a pregnant woman had intercourse with a "leper," her fetus could be infected even though the mother was not. In some cases of syphilis, the mother will show no symptoms because the disease is in remission, while the infant can be obviously sick.

and topically.[18] Over the years, some historians have pointed to these and other discrepancies as part of an attempt to prove that leprosy was syphilis. They have made similar arguments for other suggestive diseases as well.[19] But because of the strength of the Columbian hypothesis, the evidence has not been regarded as convincing. Perhaps now it can be revisited.

In addition to highlighting the unknown nature of Edward IV's disease, the anonymous Crowland chronicler claimed that it would have been difficult to cure even "in a person of lesser status" (*in minori persona*). This comment makes little sense unless we consider the possibility that Edward suffered from treponematosis, a disease unusual for having different outcomes in its endemic and venereal forms. Apparently, the chronicler was familiar enough with the disease to understand this, indicating that it was common in fifteenth-century England. As we have seen, under living conditions in which young children spend much of their time outdoors, playing together in farmyards and fields, often scantily clothed, and sharing beds and cups—that is, the living conditions of children raised as commoners—bejel would have spread easily as a childhood disease, just as it did in the modern Middle East as studied by Hudson. When people infected with bejel as children suffer a recurrence of the disease as adults, their immune systems combat it successfully and the fatality rate remains low. But this was not the case for premodern elites who contracted syphilis in adulthood. They often suffered more devastating illnesses and died young, just like Edward IV.

The existence of such a *mort mal* primarily among elites may have led to a certain degree of obfuscation in the medi-

---

18 Hudson, "Historical Approach to the Terminology of Syphilis" (1961), 548; Holcomb, "The Antiquity of Syphilis" (1935), 317–20.

19 For an introduction to this literature, see Baker and Armelagos, "The Origin and Antiquity of Syphilis" (1988), 703–7. More recently, Kaplan has argued convincingly that one such disease was *fuego persico*, discussed by Bernard Gordon in his *Lilium medicinae* (1305): Kaplan, "The (Columbian) Myth of Syphilis" (2002), 23–25.

cal literature, as kings and noblemen sought to prevent their social inferiors, contemporaries, and posterity from learning about the more terrible scourge that God had sent to punish them for their sins.[20] Still, there are hints in the historical record. The Spanish physician Gaspare Torrella (1452–1520), who treated several members of the papal court, including Cesare Borgia, wrote that in southern Spain the disease he called "*pudendagra*" was known as *morbus curialis* because of its association with the court. In eastern Europe it was called "the malady of palaces." And in France, the association of syphilis with court life was responsible for the term *mal de cour*, which usage lasted into modern times.[21] Even after widespread discussion of the new disease was facilitated by the dissemination of printed books in the early sixteenth-century, the Rouen physician Jacques de Béthencourt

---

20 The name *mort mal* is Theodoric Borgognoni's. He taught that, like *scabies grossa*, the deadly disease was a form of leprosy: Hudson, "Historical Approach to the Terminology of Syphilis" (1961), 548. Bruce Boehrer makes the point that patronage at the highest levels of the social order was responsible for the production of virtually every work on syphilis written in the first one hundred years after its appearance in Naples. He concludes that, given their provenance, "It is thus hard to avoid viewing these early texts as to some degree government documents, responsive to the needs and expectations of an aristocracy that claims its authority as God-given and immutable. In effect, when we read early texts like [Joseph] Grünpeck's with their careful appeals to patronage and their oblique echoes of theological and imperial authority, we witness the elaborate mutual fondling whereby political orthodoxies are established and maintained. The remarkable thing given this arrangement, is that any sort of effective medical study could proceed at all." See Boehrer, "Early Modern Syphilis" (1990), 205.

21 Arrizabalaga, "The Changing Identity of the French Pox" (2011), 412; Jankauskas, "Syphilis in Eastern Europe" (1994), 238. On the name "pudendagra," invented by Torrella when he observed that syphilis often appeared first in the genitalia, see Arrizabalaga, Henderson, and French, *The Great Pox* (1997), 117.

(1477–ca. 1527) observed that syphilis was still being called "the disease of the magnates" by many.[22] To have such staying power, it seems there must have been some truth in the association of syphilis with court life.

The historian Jon Arrizabalaga has investigated this question for Castile, specifically. He found a variety of opinions among medical authorities, as commonly occur in discussions of the origins and causes of syphilis. What is important for our purposes is the fact that early writers of medical treatises in Castile commented on the social status of those contracting the dangerous disease, just as the Crowland chronicler did. A physician called Francisco Núñez de la Yerva (ca. 1460–after 1504), for example, wrote that "those men accustomed to intense labor such as peasants and workers are mostly immune to this condition." By contrast, he noted that "those scarcely accustomed to work are its usual victims."[23] Núñez de la Yerva was a young doctor practising in a Leonese town, Ciudad Rodrigo, so presumably he was reporting on what he observed there. Another older and more established court physician, Juan de Fogeda (ca. 1450–after 1508), claimed the opposite, however. He said that the disease infected primarily ordinary men. Nevertheless, he aimed his advice for avoiding contagion at elites, perhaps because he wrote his treatise for Juan Téllez Girón (1456–1528), count of Ureña. As Arrizabalaga observes of Fogeda's directions, "He disapproved of violent physical exercises or movements, and advised mild exercises such as peaceful walks along smooth places, riding horses, soft massaging, or sporadic baths in fresh water: in other words, an inventory of activities perfectly fitting the regime expectations of middle-aged wealthy people like his

---

22 Major, *Classic Descriptions of Disease* (1945), 35–36, citing Béthencourt's *New Litany of Penitence* (1527). See also the sixteenth-century references cited by Holcomb, "Christopher Columbus and the American Origin of Syphilis" (1934), 11–12.

23 Quoted in Arrizabalaga, "The Changing Identity of the French Pox" (2011), 413.

master."[24] Both physicians cannot be right, so perhaps Fogeda was telling the count only what he wanted to hear. On this point, it may also be important that Núñez de la Yerva believed similar diseases to have existed in the past. He cited Pliny the Elder on mentagra, a skin disease that appeared in Rome during the reign of Tiberius Claudius. Significantly, Pliny said that mentagra affected noblemen but not commoners or servants.[25] This observation points directly to treponematosis in its endemic and venereal forms.

One final point needs to be made on the relationship between syndromes of treponematosis. A pregnant mother afflicted with syphilis can infect her child *in utero*, and congenital transmission also occurs in bejel and yaws, although less commonly. This tragic adaptation of the treponeme to its human host results in miscarriages, still births, and congenital forms of the disease in children.[26] The similarity in transmission points to the fact that all three syndromes are caused by the same microorganism, *Treponema pallidum.*[27] Only recently have scholars come to accept the so-called "unitarian" nature

---

24 Arrizabalaga, "The Changing Identity of the French Pox" (2011), 413.

25 Arrizabalaga, "The Changing Identity of the French Pox" (2011), 414.

26 The evidence is summarized in Baker et al., "Advancing the Understanding" (2020), 7, 19. Congenital treponematosis is less common in bejel and yaws, probably because by the time infected girls reach childbearing age the disease has gone into remission. See Baker et al., "Advancing the Understanding" (2020), 7, and sources there cited.

27 For an overview of the unitarian nature of treponematosis and current efforts to achieve eradication, see Giancarni and Lukehart, "The Endemic Treponematoses" (2014), 90, where they observe: "The syphilis, yaws, and bejel spirochetes were originally classified as separate species but are now considered to be subspecies of *Treponema pallidum* (*T. pallidum* subsp. *pallidum*, *T. pallidum* subsp. *pertenue*, and *T. pallidum* subsp. *endemicum*, respectively) based upon DNA hybridization evidence of their remarkably high genetic relatedness."

of treponematosis, first proposed by Hudson in 1946, to general and long-lasting skepticism.[28] According to the most recent findings, as summarized by Baker and her co-authors,

> Based upon clinical studies, genetic evidence, and research on diagnostic lesions in human skeletal remains, we conclude that syphilis, bejel (endemic syphilis), and yaws are the same disease from a pathophysiological viewpoint and are all caused by a single species, *Treponema pallidum*. All are treated today with antibiotics. We assert that their reported clinical "differences" are the result of the serendipity of transmission, age of acquisition, and variation in host response, rather than clear genetic differences in the etiological agents.[29]

The distinction between treponematosis in its venereal and endemic forms perfectly fits the statement of the Crowland chronicler, that Edward's prognosis compared unfavourably with that of a man of lesser status afflicted with the same disease. It is also highly significant that a similar statement was made about an ulcerous sore on Henry VIII's leg at the end of his life, because historians have long debated the possibility that Henry died of syphilis. As the courtier Sir Geoffrey Pole observed, "Thoughe the Kyng gloryed with the tytylle to be Supreme Hede next God, yet he had a sore lege that no pore [poor] man wold be glad off, and that he shold not lyve long for all his auctoryte next God."[30] Both kings, it seems, had a disease found among their

---

28 Hudson, "A Unitarian View of Treponematosis" (1946); and Hudson, "The Treponematoses—or Treponematosis?" (1958).

29 See Baker et al., "Advancing the Understanding" (2020), 28. The fourth treponemal disease, pinta, remains unclassified. Baker and colleagues observe (8): "Because there is no extant isolate from pinta, there is no genetic information; thus, its relationship to *T. pallidum* is unknown. Its causative agent, therefore, is still called *T. carateum.*"

30 *Letters and Papers*, ed. Gairdner, 13.2:313. Henry probably suffered from a painful gummatous lesion typical of tertiary syphilis.

subjects and yet more difficult to cure when it appeared at court. Syphilis fits this description.

Let us turn now to a second obscure comment on the death of Edward IV, one made by the Italian visitor Mancini, for it corroborates this interpretation and allows us to enter the realm of medieval attitudes toward venereal disease. After reporting that some people believed the king was depressed over the failure of his foreign policy, Mancini says that Edward fell victim to a cold on what was apparently a very exciting fishing expedition.

> So as to raise or disguise this sorrow of his, in those days Edward produced many entertainments and theatrical spectacles with royal splendor, although he was never entirely able to conceal it. Indeed, to this sadness of his they [my sources] add that the man was of extreme height and certainly quite fat, although not to the point of deformity, so that when on a certain day he himself sailed a boat with those whom he had ordered to go fishing, and watched the fishing quite avidly, he received a damp chill to his very marrow. From this, he was seized by a disease from which he did not recover, and was afflicted even further.[31]

Although specific in its details, Mancini's statement was not meant to be taken literally. It is my contention that in late medieval Europe "fishing" was a euphemism for the physical

---

For a detailed description of various manifestations of tertiary gumma in the skin, subcutaneous tissue, muscle, and bone, see Mraček, *Atlas of Syphilis* (1898), 30–38.

31 Mancini, *Usurpation*, ed. and trans. Armstrong, 59; this translation is by Carol Symes. The Latin reads: "Ad dolorem vero ipsum levandum vel dissimulandum etsi iisdiebus Eduardus multos ludos cum scenicis et regiis apparatibus editerit, nunquam tamen omnino accultare potuit. Huic tristitie et illud adiungunt, quod homo procere stature, maximeque pinguis non tamen ad defromitatem, cum quadum die et ipse navicula vectus, cum iis quos piscari iusserat, avidius piscationem spectasset, humidum frigus ad medullas admisit. Unde eo morbo correptus est, a quo non convaluit, nec diu afflictus fuit."

act of intercourse, a symbolism that historians have not yet fully understood. So, when the humanist scholar Erasmus of Rotterdam (1466–1536), who loved wordplay, remarked that Guiliano della Rovere, later pope Julius II, spent his youth rowing the fishing boat of his father, he was probably referring to the pope's immoral sexual behaviour, not his occupation, for it was widely known that Julius suffered from syphilis.[32] In telling his fishing story, Mancini was engaging in a similarly indirect critique of the English king. Edward, it seems, had not gone fishing at all but participated in, or at least watched, some kind of group sexual activity, perhaps on the water.

Evidence for such a startling conjecture comes from the study of piscatorial symbolism by art historian Eddy de Jongh, who observes that fish have been given erotic connotations since antiquity. "Fish were to be granted a long life as phallic and fertility symbols, to which they were elevated already in the earliest days of human civilization. The Italian word for fish, *pesce*, was used regionally to indicate the male member, and in Turkish vernacular the penis is known as a 'one-eyed fish'."[33] To De Jongh's linguistic examples we can add others. The Old French and Anglo-Norman words for "fisher" (*pescheor/pecheur*) and "sinner" (*pecheur/pechour*) are similar, while the English word for the pocket-like covering that fit over the genitals otherwise exposed by men's hose was "codpiece."[34] It may have derived its name from the "cod" in a fishing net, the gathering at the bottom to prevent the fish from escaping, or more probably (as cod was a synonym for "bag") both terms came from the "cod"

---

32 Erasmus, *Adages*, trans. Drysdall, 53. See also *The Julius Exclusus*, 50–51 and 111–12nn17–18. On this point, we should remember that the pope came from a prominent family, not one that would have required him to perform manual labour as a fisherman. On the pope's health, see Arrizabalaga, Henderson, and French, *The Great Pox* (1997), 113.

33 De Jongh, "Symbolism of Fish," 102, 110.

34 I would like to thank Carol Symes for her help with the Old French and Anglo-Norman vocabulary.

or skin covering the testicles. "Codding" also meant "lecherous" or "lustful."

A vivid illuminated manuscript from the thirteenth century also suggests that there was a symbolic relationship between fishing and the physical act of intercourse in medieval France. In it, we see a pair of lovers embracing in a bed surrounded by curtains painted in the shape of two large fish tails. One of the tails joins seamlessly with the woman's netted hair, which is painted in the same colors as though it were an extension of the tail.[35] Accompanying text from *Le Régime du corps* by Aldobrandino of Siena (d. 1296 or 1299) advises couples on how to conceive a healthy child. The smiles on the faces of this married pair indicate they may be enjoying their sexual encounter too much for the good of their souls, however, for the Church taught that intercourse was designed by God not to give pleasure, but for procreation alone. Although clearly intended by God, intercourse had been irretrievably tainted by the loss of prelapsarian purity, and sexual relations could never be as pure as God had designed them to be because of Original Sin. All that remained was to attempt to limit sin, to enjoy sexual pleasure as an effect of intercourse, not a motivator: a venial sin, not a mortal one.[36] According to James A. Brundage, "Several influential canonists taught that sexual pleasure was a result of original sin and hence that the enjoyment of sex, even in marriage, was irretrievably tainted with sin. [...] The only exception was intercourse for the purpose of reproduction, and even in that situation some canonists thought that the pleasure derived from the experience was wrong."[37] If sexual desire, pleasure, and gratification held the risk of sin even within marriage, then outside of conjugal relations intercourse was regarded as supremely dangerous to the soul. The association of fishing with illicit intercourse was therefore particularly strong.

---

35 As noted by Camille, "Manuscript Illumination," 62.

36 Payer provides an illuminating discussion of Thomas Aquinas' views on this point in his *The Bridling of Desire*, 161–81.

37 Brundage, "Concubinage and Marriage," 4.

An example of "fishing" as a euphemism for intercourse comes from a period that scholars know was plagued by syphilis, and so speaks directly to the meaning of Mancini's comment on the cause of Edward IV's death. In his *Bulwarke of Defence Againste All Sicknes, Sornes, and Woundes* (1562), the physician William Bullein advised his readers to use the guaiacum cure for syphilis, but warned that it was not to be undertaken lightly. "Many men have written moche of this Poxe, after sondry sortes, and divers waies, and have killed not a fewe with long diattes, but I will speake that, whiche I do knowe, proved and seen, to have helped very many. Yet would I not, *that any should fishe for this disease*, or be to bold when he is bitten, to think hereby to be helped: but rather eschue the cause of this infirmitie, and filthy, rotten, burning of harlottes, etc."[38]

Probably more than any other imagery, the mermaid exemplifies the association of women with sexual sin, for the lower half of her body is turned completely into a fish and she is invariably shown with her hair down and breasts bared. Frequently, she stares brazenly at the viewer in full frontal pose, even when carved in church misericords or roof bosses. Illuminations from medieval religious books show mermaids tempting sailors at sea or pulling them aggressively into the water, while mermaids with two tails held apart in a come-hither gesture show their desire for intercourse with the viewer. That such graphic images of the mermaid as temptress appeared in churches and devotional books indicates they were used to remind Christians of the danger to their souls of sexual sin.[39] Mermaid imagery seems therefore to have been meant as a warning to men about the physical

---

38 Quoted in Fabricius, *Syphilis in Shakespeare's England*, 70 (emphasis added). Guaiacum, comprising several species of flowering shrubs and trees native to the Americas, provided the wood used to make a drug employed in treating syphilis in early modern Europe.

39 Betcher discusses traditional mermaid iconography in "A Tempting Theory," 65–66. She focuses on mermaids as temptresses who seek to lure sailors to watery deaths, noting that in the Christian era mermaids were associated with the devil because they lacked

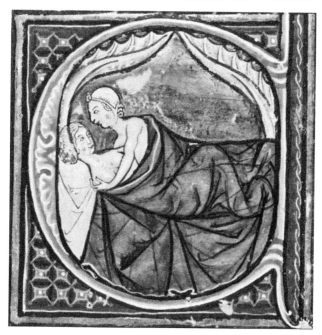

Figure 1. Fishtail bed curtains illustrate medieval attitudes toward sexual intercourse: from a late thirteenth-century manuscript illumination. Northern France, ca. 1285. London, British Library, MS Sloane 2435, fol. 9v. © British Library Board.

danger of intercourse with women, whose faces and breasts could be beautiful while the lower part of their bodies—the mysterious genitalia—might prove menacing.

After contracting syphilis, a woman often shows no symptoms of the disease in the primary and most infectious stage because the chancre that is the site of infection is usually internal. She also does not know she has syphilis at this stage,

souls. Bennett writes that mermaid imagery was "everywhere" in late medieval England: "Death and the Maiden," 281–82.

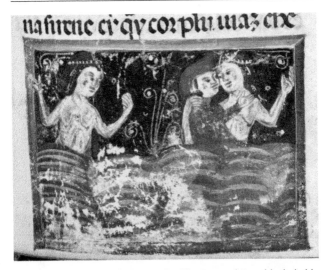

na firene ci qy cor plu maz cic

Figure 2. Mermaids, called sirens in this manuscript and included in a chapter titled "On Animals," tempt a man to engage in sex. This version of Anglicus's influential treatise has unusually detailed pictorial representations of disease, some pointing to symptoms of syphilis under other names. Bartholomaeus Anglicus, *On the Properties of Things*, Italy, ca. 1309. London, British Library, MS Additional 8785, fol. 298. © British Library Board.

because the chancre is painless.[40] In the case of a man, the situation is different, because the primary lesion is visible on the penis. A story told by the fourteenth-century travel writer Sir John Mandeville, a pseudonym, is useful for demonstrating that some people believed women could unknowingly give men a fatal disease during intercourse. "Mandeville" writes that he visited an island where newly married men allowed other men to have intercourse with their brides before daring

---

40 For an introduction to medieval medical ideas about the physical danger to men of intercourse with women, see Álvarez and Rodriguez, "Moral Considerations," 55–57.

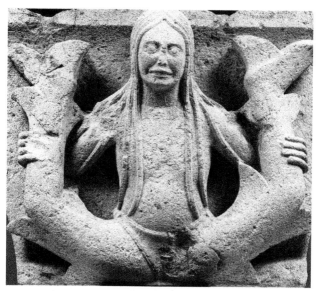

Figure 3. Sculpted by Wiligelmo da Modena (fl. ca. 1099–1120) as part of a decorative motif for the Duomo di Modena, this fork-tailed mermaid has feet visible in her tail fins that emphasize the conflation of women with fish. © Lapidary Museum, Modena, Italy © Evelyn Aschenbrenner, 2010.

to do so themselves. "And I asked what was their cause why they did so, and they said some husbands lay by their wives and none other but they, and some of their wives had snakes in their bodies that stung their husbands upon their penises in the bodies of the women, and so was many a man slain."[41] In what is clearly an apocryphal tale, men who were fearful of

---

41 Quoted in Bennett, "Death and the Maiden," 282–83. The Middle English version reads, "And Y askyd what was here cause wei þei dide so, and þei seide somme housbandis lay by here wyfes and none oþer but þei, and somme of here wyfes hadde naddris in here bodyes þat twengid here housbandis upon here ȝerdys in

dying wanted to make sure their new wives were snake-free, or what is more likely, disease-free, before lying with them. This would seem to indicate an understanding of the connection between intercourse and the deadly "serpentine disease."[42]

The *Bible moralisée* contained in Österreichische Nationalbibliothek, Codex Vindobonensis 2554, an illustrated Bible from the thirteenth century, highlights the connection between certain kinds of fish and sexual sin. It shows images from Leviticus in which Moses instructs the Jewish people to eat fish with scales such as pike and salmon, but not eels or tench that are smooth. The instruction in the accompanying text is moral, warning, "The eel which is slippery signifies the woman who is deceptive and who can neither be held nor known. The tench signifies those who live in lust and covetousness."[43] Similarly, the historian Marcel Thomas tells us, in a discussion of a marginal painting in a fifteenth-century devotional manuscript, *The Rohan Book of Hours*, that the tench is compared to "filth," or sexual relations with prostitutes. He further notes, of an image included to illustrate one of the biblical texts on Jewish dietary laws, that it shows a man tempted by "two unsavory women, who have already been compared to the eel and the tench."[44] The tench is a fish with very small scales and a thick skin, making it as slippery as an eel, hence the comparison. By distinguishing between

---

þe bodyes of þe wymmen, and so was many a man yslawe." See Mandeville, *The Defective Version*, ed. Seymour, 122–23.

42 For an introduction to the question of the text's authorship see M. C. Seymour, "Mandeville, Sir John," in the *Oxford Dictionary of National Biography*. Seymour notes that Jean d'Outremeuse of Liège, a chronicler and notary, claimed that a physician of his city, Jean de Bourgogne, had been the author of Mandeville's manuscript. This has since been proven false, but it is quite possible that the snake story came from a physician familiar with symptoms of the "serpentine disease," if not from Bourgogne himself.

43 *Bible Moralisée*, trans. Guest, 86.

44 *Rohan Book of Hours*, intro. Meiss and Thomas, commentary on plates 99, 101.

fish representing morality and immorality, the commentator kept the ever-present possibility of sexual sin on the minds of his readers.

The English in particular seem to have used eel symbolism in works of art, as seen in a startling and highly unusual stained-glass window from Great Malvern Priory that shows a large conger eel slithering between the feet of St. John the Baptist. It had been thought that the head was part of the traditional camel hair tunic of St. John (barely visible here beneath the white robe), but the association of fish, and especially eels, with sexual sin means we can now see that the head is indeed that of an eel.[45] Certainly, it fulfills the important role of creating great unease in the viewer. Also in this church is a window with a scene showing the Last Supper. The traditional meal of lamb has been replaced by one of pickerel. In front of the table sits Judas opening his mouth to take the communion wafer offered to him by Christ. At the same time, Judas lifts the tablecloth to give the viewer a good look at a fish (or possibly an eel given its long, thin body and large round eye) that is curled in his lap. The traditional conjecture that Judas is stealing a fish to remind viewers of his thievish nature does not quite fit the occasion, as he is about to betray Christ, making it unlikely he is thinking about his next meal. Once again we see fish symbolism being used to represent sinful humanity, this time in the person of Judas.[46] It was a connection stained-glass artists working in Worcestershire seem to have believed the congregation would understand.

---

45 Rather than a scalped camel, as Rushforth proposed: *Medieval Christian Imagery*, 234.

46 Rushforth, *Medieval Christian Imagery*, 61–63. On the meal of fish, Rushforth writes that it was "a survival of the primitive symbolical representation of the Eucharist in the Catacomb art by fish, loaves, and a vessel of wine, the former being an allusion to the miracle of the loaves and fishes (Mark vi, &c.) as a type of the sacrament."

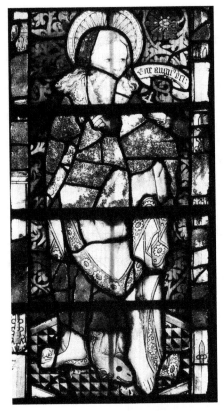

Figure 4. St. John the Baptist's conger eel. Great Malvern Priory, Malvern, Worcestershire, fifteenth century. © Katherine Little, 2021.

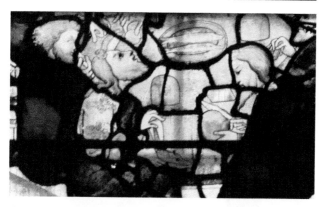

Figure 5. Judas hiding a fish or eel: detail from "The Last Supper." Great Malvern Priory, Malvern, Worcestershire, fifteenth century. © Katherine Little, 2021.

Medieval churches frequently have wall paintings of St. Christopher that show a variety of fish—sometimes including mermaids—swimming about the saint's feet, while eels twine around his staff or legs.[47] Eleanor Pridgeon, a close student of the genre, has counted two hundred and six St. Christopher wall paintings that survive in churches in England and Wales, among many more that have been lost. They usually appear in the nave, an area of the church reserved for lessons

---

[47] For a detailed discussion of St. Christopher artworks that include mermaids, see Hernando Garrido, "San Cristóbal y la Sirenita." He argues that mermaids were perceived as temptresses, particularly for travellers, which he believes can explain their association with Christopher even in inland mountainous areas populated primarily by shepherds and their flocks. He notes (264) that, in the sixteenth and seventeenth centuries, prostitutes were sometimes called mermaids. Betcher also sees the mermaids in St. Christopher wall paintings as temptresses, and argues they were meant to remind the viewer that Christopher had resisted temptation by prostitutes in prison and converted them to Christianity: see "A Tempting Theory," 68.

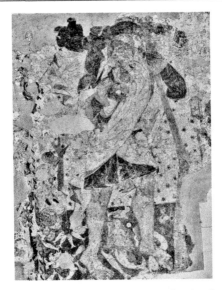

Figure 6. Although the upper half of this medieval wall painting is heavily damaged, we can still see St. Christopher striding across the river with his heavenly burden. Around his feet swim a wide variety of well-preserved fish, some about to be caught by an angler, and a mermaid with long, golden hair who gazes at herself appreciatively in a mirror. The saint crushes a large eel with his foot, symbolizing the power of God to conquer evil. All Saints Church, Oaksey, Wiltshire. © James Meakin, 2021.

on morality, which may explain the presence of so many fish, especially eels, in the paintings.[48] *The Golden Legend* (ca. 1260) by Jacobus de Voragine (1228/30–1298), a source for much of what late medieval Christians knew about Christopher, says

---

48 Pridgeon, "Saint Christopher Wall Paintings," 111 and 128–29. According to Katherine Little, an authority on the stained-glass windows of Great Malvern Priory, the window showing an eel between the feet of John the Baptist (Figure 4) was originally located in the nave.

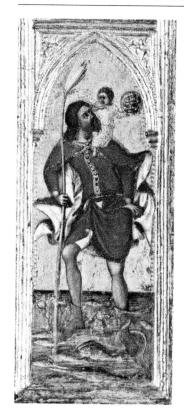

Figure 7. An eel curls around the leg of St. Christopher and his feet are surrounded with a variety of sea creatures, including an octopus, in a detail from a richly painted triptych. Madonna of Humility (detail), ca. 1370–1375 by Niccolò di Buonaccorso. Putnam Foundation, Timken Museum of Art, San Diego, CA.

that he was a giant who converted to Christianity after seeking the most powerful man on earth in order to serve in his retinue—and discovering that he was Jesus.[49] The story most

---

49 According to Eamon Duffy, *The Golden Legend* was compiled to provide priests with material to use in their sermons. It became extremely popular, "surviving in nearly one thousand Latin manuscripts and five hundred translations in a variety of European vernaculars." See his introduction to Jacobus de Voragine, *The Golden Legend*, trans. Ryan, xi. For the life of St. Christopher, see 396–400.

closely associated with the saint, and the one invariably portrayed in English parish churches and many other European artworks, depicts him carrying the Christ child on his shoulder while crossing a river, often teeming with fish. Christopher does not recognize the child who has asked for his help, but as he walks his burden becomes almost unbearably heavy. When they reach the opposite riverbank Christ tells the saint that the great weight came from carrying the whole world on his shoulders, along with the God who created it.

Pridgeon believes that the prominence of St. Christopher wall paintings in English and Welsh churches can be explained by the presence of an "image-based cult" of the saint in the late fifteenth-century. It focused on the belief that, if a person saw Christopher's image, they would not suffer from misadventure or die a sudden or ill death that day.[50] The saint's protective function was invoked in prayer as well, for *The Golden Legend* says that Christopher "besought your forgiveness and by his supplications obtained the cure of diseases and infirmities." Pridgeon further notes that the English printer William Caxton makes a change to this wording in his translation of *The Golden Legend*, which he printed in Westminster between November 1483 and March 1484: "and he also gat of thee by prayer power to put away sickness and sores from them that remember his passion and figure."[51] As Pridgeon observes, Caxton "may have recognised that St. Christopher functioned as a healer in imagery, and he may have modified the saintly functions to ensure his text was reflective of practice and belief in fifteenth-century society. Caxton certainly made additions elsewhere, supplementing the text with some sixty saints of his own, and inserting his own words where he felt it necessary."[52] In addition to the possibility that Caxton understood the importance of St. Christopher as a

---

50 Pridgeon, "Saint Christopher Wall Paintings," 94–95.

51 Jacobus de Voragine, *The Golden Legend [...] as Englished by William Caxton*, 119.

52 Pridgeon, "Saint Christopher Wall Paintings," 98.

healer, his mention of a single symptom of disease—sores—is suggestive: they are a prominent symptom of both acquired and congenital syphilis, which may have been prevalent in late medieval England. Perhaps, then, it was fear of syphilis in particular that prompted elites to include wall paintings and stained-glass windows of Christopher in their churches, and illuminations of the saint in their books of hours.

Textual evidence that this was the case comes from an early fourteenth-century St. Christopher wall painting in the Church of the Holy Rood in Woodeaton, Oxfordshire. It shows an octopus between the saint's legs among a variety of fish, but its most important feature is the long scroll descending from the figure of the Christ child. In Pridgeon's translation, it tells the viewer that seeing the saint's image will provide protection from an "ill death" that day. ("Ki cest image verra le jur de male mort ne murra"—Whoever sees this image will not suffer an ill death [*male mort*] today.)[53] But the word "ill" may not be strong enough for what people were experiencing in Oxfordshire. Now that we know treponematosis existed in premodern Europe, it seems possible the saint's protection extended to the venereal form of that disease in particular, for the words *male mort* reversed (*mort male*, or deadly disease) appeared in a highly influential surgical treatise by the Italian bishop Theodoric Borgognoni (1205–1296), specifically in reference to a form of "leprosy" that could be cured with mercury.[54] As previously noted, Hansen's Disease cannot be treated with mercury, but syphilis can.

Within the context of the symbolic meaning of fish and fishing, the curious statement by Mancini—that Edward IV died after fishing with companions on the Thames—indicates that some courtiers believed the king to have died from complications of a sexually transmitted disease. The disease was almost certainly syphilis, a progressive illness that would

---

53 Pridgeon, "Saint Christopher Wall Paintings," 94.

54 Hudson, "Historical Approach to the Terminology of Syphilis" (1961), 548.

have been visible to those surrounding the king for years before his death. This also fits a statement by another contemporary, that the king's illness "continued longer than false and fantasticall tales have untruly and falsely surmised, as I myself that wrote this pamphlet truly knew."[55] It also accords with a comment in the records of the city of Canterbury, dating from 1481 or 1482, in which the mayor reported that William, Lord Hastings, a close adviser to the king throughout his reign, told the mayor that the king's health was not good.[56] In the tertiary stage, syphilis can affect not only the nervous system but also the arteries, which makes a heart attack or stroke more likely even in young sufferers.[57]

One final piece of evidence that Edward may have had syphilis lies in the possibility that his younger son, Richard duke of York, inherited the disease from his parents. It is perhaps significant that a man claiming to be the younger son of Edward IV, Richard duke of York, may have suffered from a common symptom of congenital syphilis, interstitial keratitis, which leads to clouding of the cornea. In 1496, the officer of arms known as Richmond Herald (Roger Machado?) told the ambassador to the duke of Milan, Raimondo de Soncino, that this man "is not handsome, indeed his left eye rather lacks luster." The delayed appearance of interstitial keratitis in later childhood or adolescence could then explain the confusion of the Spanish knight Rui de Sousa, who testified that a man he saw in Portugal, reputed to be York, could not (he reasoned) be the same person because the young duke had been "very beautiful" as a child—"the most beautiful creature he had ever seen"—while this man was not. It was

---

55 *Chronicle of John Hardyng*, ed. Ellis, 470. Henry Ellis, in his introduction (xx), posits that the author of the statement, as recorded by Grafton in his continuation of the chronicle, was John Morton archbishop of Canterbury.

56 Ross, *Edward IV*, 287n3.

57 Holcomb refers to studies of cardiovascular disease in syphilis showing rates of heart involvement of 70–80 percent and 86.3–97.6 percent: "The Antiquity of Syphilis" (1935), 311.

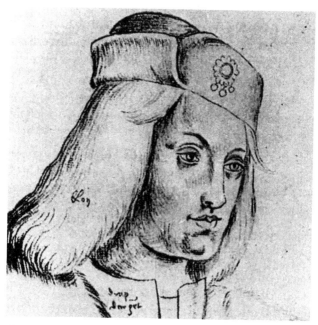

Figure 8. Richard duke of York (1473-?) was the second son of Edward IV and his queen Elizabeth Woodville. He may be the man depicted here in a drawing by the sixteenth-century French artist Jacques Le Boucq copied from a contemporary portrait, perhaps as part of a series created for the Holy Roman Emperor, Charles V. There is some similarity of features to the portrait of Edward IV owned by the Society of Antiquaries. From the *Recueil d'Arras*. Media Arras, MS no. 266, fol. 23.

probably the diseased eye that made the man de Sousa saw unattractive in adulthood. This conjecture fits a diagnosis of interstitial keratitis if the man were the real Richard duke of York, whose father died of syphilis and who might, therefore, have had congenital syphilis, and not the imposter whom Henry VII called Perkin Warbeck. A drawing of the mature duke, attributed to Jacques le Boucq, provides corroborating evidence. It shows a man with a left eye that has no highlight, indicating opacity or perhaps blindness, and a drooping eye-lid (ptosis), symptoms of congenital syphilis.[58]

If Edward IV did die of syphilis, it would help to explain a reported scene in which Richard, duke of Gloucester (later Richard III), and Henry Stafford, duke of Buckingham, informed the king's son, Edward V, that his father's death had been caused by his evil companions. According to an account of their conversation by Mancini, "They exhibited a mournful countenance, while expressing profound grief at the death of the king's father whose demise they imputed to his ministers as being such that they had but little regard for his honour, since they were accounted the companions and servants of his vices, and had ruined his health."[59] Death from a sexually transmitted disease fits this statement better than death from overeating and drinking. In the end, despite his lifetime of indulgences, Edward reportedly died repentant. If true, his contrition must have been a great relief to his spiritual advisers, for it now appears he had died of an illness that was highly disturbing to his contemporaries.

---

58 Wroe, *The Perfect Prince*, 9–10, 525–26. *Calendar of State Papers and Manuscripts Existing in the Archives and Collections of Milan*, ed. Hinds (1912), 330. On drooping eyelids in congenital syphilis see Hutchinson, *Syphilis* (1910): 306–8.

59 Mancini, *Usurpation*, ed. and trans. Armstrong, 77. "Deinde de obitu patris in corde dolorem in vultu tristitiam ostendunt, cuius mortem eius administris imputant: quia qui parum eius honori consuluissent, cum libidinum socii et structores haberentur, eiusdem etiam salute precipitassent."

Chapter 3

Evidence from Medical Writings: A Suggestive Example

Given what we now know about the existence of treponematosis in the premodern world, it will be necessary to reexamine ancient and medieval medical treatises that might yield evidence of the disease. Two clinicians-turned-historians of the twentieth century, Ellis Herndon Hudson and Richmond C. Holcomb, have led the way and their provocative findings need to be reconsidered, along with those of other historians who remained skeptical of the Columbian hypothesis. In addition, much original work will have to be undertaken to create a fuller picture. Such an endeavour is beyond the scope of this study, but examples from the writings of one man, John Arderne (b. 1307/8, d. in or after 1377), may serve to highlight the need for careful analytical work in these rich sources.

Arderne was a respected general surgeon, best known for his treatment of anal fistulas, for which he pioneered a number of highly effective techniques.[1] He was proud of his success, which brought him wealth and fame. He tells us, in his *Practica*, that he charged £40 (forty pounds) for his ser-

---

1 An anal fistula can occur when a mucus-producing gland inside the anus becomes infected and develops into an abscess. Left untreated, a small tunnel develops that opens in the skin near the anus. An abscess on the buttocks can produce a fistula when it grows internally until it perforates the anus or rectum. Fistulas also occur when an ulcer on the wall of the rectum, colon, or bladder perforates and connects with the vagina or uterus.

vices, an extraordinary amount for the era. As observed by Peter Murray Jones, the foremost expert on Arderne:

> The very fact that Arderne thought that these operations constituted his claim to fame is somewhat surprising, given that the condition of fistula-in-ano is not normally regarded today as life-threatening, nor is it particularly prevalent in the populations of either developed or developing countries. D'Arcy Power speculated about the effect of long hours spent in the saddle in unpleasant weather by knights in the Hundred Years' War—in any event it seems that Arderne found sufficient patients willing to elect surgery and to pay his huge fees.[2]

These fees are commensurate with the elevated status of Arderne's patients.[3] Based on recent discoveries, we can now posit that the need for anal surgery was a consequence of the prevalence of syphilis among elites in Arderne's day. One common symptom of the secondary stage of the disease is *condyloma lata*, lesions that appear around the anus. As described by the nineteenth-century syphilologist Franz Mraček, "In the anal region peculiar formations sometimes develop on account of the anatomical parts. The folds become longer, hard, and infiltrated; the intervals between them are marked by deep fissures which penetrate into the aperture of the anus."[4] Fissures that were so deep and serious they could turn into fistulas would explain Arderne's interest in this area of medicine, including his decision to write a medical treatise focusing on a single type of surgery, which was unusual for the era.[5] Supporting this conjecture is Jones's

---

2 Peter Murray Jones, "Arderne, John," in the *Oxford Dictionary of National Biography*.

3 Jones, "John of Arderne," 296. D'Arcy Power describes Arderne's patients as "chiefly knights and priests, sometimes citizens, occasionally ladies": "Lesser Writings," 132. See also Turner, "Thomas Usk and John Arderne," 100–101.

4 Mraček, *Atlas of Syphilis* (1898), 25.

5 Jones, "Four Middle English Translations," 65–66. Arderne's

discovery that "much of Arderne's practice was taken up with the visible ailments affecting the limbs of his patients, while the number of cases affecting the male genitalia hint at something of a specialism."[6]

With this possibility in mind, the careful attention Arderne gave to the illustration of his works—Jones says he devised them himself—becomes significant, because one image in the *Liber medicinarum* is highly suggestive of syphilis. It shows a tonsured cleric lifting his robe to reveal his diseased penis (London, British Library, MS Sloane 56, fol. 85v). Jones tells us that Arderne meant the five precisely placed red circles to represent sores leaking urine—penile fistulas.[7] They are an indication that the penis is in an advanced state of disintegration. This image calls to mind the claim of the cleric and Oxford administrator Thomas Gascoigne (1404–1458), who wrote that John of Gaunt, duke of Lancaster (1340–1399)—one of Arderne's younger contemporaries—"died of putrefaction of his genitals and body, caused by the frequenting of women, for he was a great fornicator."[8] Gascoigne's comment has long been discredited by historians, despite evidence

---

treatise on anal fistulas was reproduced frequently both in Latin and Middle English. Jones notes that forty manuscripts survive from the period before 1600.

6 Jones, "John of Arderne," 300. Modern medical studies have revealed that ulcers and gummas of the anus, rectum, and colon are symptomatic of syphilis. For an overview, see Weisenberg, "Syphilis" (2020). See also Hollings, "Syphilitic Ulcers of the Anus" (1961), 730–31. Case reports include Bari, "Early Syphilis Presenting as Anal Fissure" (2005); Cox, "Syphilis as an Atypical Cause of Perianal Fissure" (2018).

7 Jones, "Staying with the Program," 207. Although this manuscript was created after Arderne's death, Jones argues that the program of illustrations he had created "remained remarkably resistant to change" and that the image appears as he would have wanted it to (205).

8 Gascoigne, *Loci e libro veritatum*, ed. Rogers (1881), 137: "Magnum etiam dux in Anglia, scilicet J. de Gawnt, mortuus est ex tali

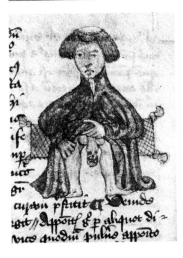

Figure 9. John Arderne, *Liber medicinarum*. England, first quarter of the fifteenth century. London, British Library, MS Sloane 56, fol. 85v. © British Library Board.

that Gaunt's son, Henry IV (1367–1413) may also have died of syphilis.[9] Perhaps now this testimony will carry more weight.

Arderne's successful and lucrative career might have resulted from treating syphilitic rashes and sores as well as

---

putrefactione membronum genitalium et corporis sui, causata per frequentationem mulierem."

9 In 1935, Griffith Davies argued that Gaunt probably had syphilis, and that his son Henry IV died from complications of congenital syphilis: Davies, *Henry V*, 4, 8, 112–14. In 1985, Peter McNiven disagreed with this diagnosis, largely because he accepted the Columbian theory: "The Problem of Henry IV's Health," 750–51. Nevertheless, McNiven's detailed and thorough discussion of Henry's declining health (768–70), beginning in 1405 and including evidence of "a sudden malady in his leg" that made it impossible for him to ride or go on campaign, as well as circulatory problems leading to strokes, is highly suggestive of tertiary syphilis, as is the desire of his council that he abdicate in favour of his son. Perhaps the fact that Davies lived in an era when syphilis was a disease of major concern helped him accept the possibility that a medieval king had died of it.

fistulas, judging from a comment he made about his cure for a disease he called "scabies." He recommended mixing mercury with the yolk of a raw egg and making it into a poultice, noting that this treatment was highly effective if the remedy were kept in place for at least thirty, and preferably forty, days. "The weche I have provyd ane hundryd tymes & therwith have gote moche lucre, pro certo and that xx sol for oo lyzste (twenty shillings for one dressing)."[10] Mercury was used as a treatment for a variety of skin ailments, but it seems unlikely that any medieval physician could earn so large a sum for treating common and nonthreatening skin complaints. Fear of syphilis, however, might have prompted well-to-do patients to open their purses generously, and of course mercury was also the standard treatment for symptoms of that disease in the early sixteenth century. The need for Arderne's treatments elsewhere on the body is further exemplified by the title of a later compendium of his works, *A tretis extracte of Maistre John Arden of fistula in ano and of fistula in other place of the body and of apostemes makyng fistules and of emoraides & tenasmon and of clisteres* (ulcers causing fistulas, hemorrhoids and anal growths, and clysters).

A final hint that Arderne may have been well acquainted with symptoms of syphilis concerns advice he gave to pregnant women and nurses. Immediately preceding his discussion of scabies, Arderne includes a brief discussion of parsley as a medicinal herb that points to an understanding of congenital syphilis. "Women with child using Ache [an alternative name for parsley] engender pustules and stinking sores in the body of the child. And therefore physicians forbid women with child and nurses that keep young sucking children from Ache lest the child be made unwise or foolish therethrough."[11]

---

10 Power, "Lesser Writings," 118. Ulcers and fistulas were closely related in Arderne's mind. Jones writes that the surgeon believed fistulas to develop from *apostemata* (ulcers), explaining how they could be managed to avoid fistulation: "John of Arderne," 310–11.

11 Power, "Lesser Writings," 118 and 130. The original, from London, British Library, MS Sloane 2002, reads "Wommene with chylde

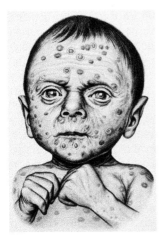

Figure 10. An infant born in 1897 with congenital syphilis, shown at four weeks. The diagnosis reads, "Marasmus marked. Suffering from bronchitis and intestinal catarrh. The skin is pale and wrinkled, and thickly covered with a syphilitic eruption. The forehead and mouth, and also the trunk and extremities, are the seat of papules and pale-red border, or vesicles containing a small quantity of serous exudate, with flaccid, partly degenerated epidermis." Mraček, *Atlas of Syphilis* (1898), plate 58. Wellcome Collection.

In large quantities, parsley does have uterotonic properties, but no ability to produce skin lesions in a fetus or to foster intellectual disabilities in a young child; syphilis, however, can do both. How women actually used parsley, whether ingesting it or making it into poultices, needs further investigation; but it appears from Arderne's remark that there was a perceived relationship between its use and the appearance of typical symptoms of congenital syphilis in infants and children. In any event, Arderne wanted to alert his readers to the connection.

Marion Turner has written about Arderne in her study of illness narratives, and she notes a tendency in the medieval period to use fistulas as a metaphor for sin. "Although Arderne is writing about actual fistulas in his tract, he is writing in an environment in which fistulas were sometimes recognized

---

usynge Ache engendryth postemys & stynkynge bocchys in the body of the chylde. And therefore lechys forfenden wommene with chylde & norycys that kepen Yonge soowkynge childerne from Ache leste that the childe be made unwise or folyssch therthorough." Power notes that Arderne had "a sound knowledge of herbs and was a great pharmacist."

as metaphors and in which illness more generally was often viewed as representing a different kind of problem, a moral problem."[12] Turner's point may have been more relevant than she understood, for if preachers often expounded from the pulpit on the spiritual meaning of disease, there may also have been a practical reason for doing so—the presence of syphilis in the population. Therefore, when Pope Innocent III (ca. 1160–1216) wrote that "sickness of the body may sometimes be the result of sin," and instituted the requirement that patients confess before undergoing surgical treatments, it was for good reason.[13] Sexual promiscuity was probably regularly producing symptoms of disease in the genitalia, anus, and rectum that could prove fatal, endangering victims' souls. Evidence that preachers and congregants were facing this reality alongside physicians comes from the use of metaphors equating spiritual death with diseased bodies in sermons of the period. Jeremy J. Citrome has studied this literature in detail and he concludes: "To the profoundly penitential culture of later medieval England, sin and sickness were inextricably linked; and surgery, even as it progressed in its ability to cure physical affliction, became even more important as a metaphor for the pursuit of spiritual health."[14]

Alongside the sermon literature and works by Arderne, Citrome has studied two poems written in the fourteenth century, the homiletic *Cleanness* and the history/romance *The Siege of Jerusalem*. In the process, he uncovered intriguing references to disease that may indicate the presence of syphilis, characterized by its filthy sores, rotting flesh, and stench. One example from *Cleanness* will suffice to introduce the possibility: the attack of the Sodomites on the gatehouse

---

12 Turner, "Illness Narratives," 64.

13 Quoted in Citrome, *The Surgeon*, 4. The new requirements for confession came out of the Fourth Lateran Council, convened by Innocent III in 1215.

14 For an illuminating discussion of this idea, see Citrome's introduction to *The Surgeon*, "Surgery and the Wounds of Sin," 1–18 (quotation at 1).

of Lot in an attempt to violate his visitors. When Lot refuses them entry, the Sodomites seek a way in, but "[t]hay lest of Lotes logging [lodging] any lysoun [lesion] to fynde" (1. 887). The use of the word "lesion" here is odd, and the translation by Citrome is based on his understanding of how the anonymous author—who was fascinated by medical literature—employed disease imagery in the poem. As he explains, "This 'lysoun' can be seen as a distinctly corporeal image. The healthy body is often presented in medieval medical writings as enclosed, without lesions. [...] Lesions, in the physiological sense, are openings in the flesh, and in the Middle Ages they were thought to signal the beginnings of an ulcerate wound. [...] Ulcers, then, are a fitting metaphor for the blemishes, caused by moral corruption, which must be excised from the soul."[15] With Citrome's work as a guide, it appears that poetry and romances, as well as sermons, could reveal a wealth of information on the existence of syphilis in the medieval world, just as the medical treatises appear to do.

---

15 Citrome, *The Surgeon*, 25.

Chapter 4

Evidence from Illuminated Manuscripts, Stained Glass, and Paintings

While it is clear that a dramatic outbreak of syphilis occurred in Naples at the end of the fifteenth century, making that disease newly visible because of its virulence, paleopathologists have now proved that treponematosis existed in the Old World previous to that famous epidemic. It has therefore become important to re-examine not only documentary sources but also visual ones for evidence of the venereal form of that disease. These sources may help to document the extent of syphilis in Europe, where it seems to have been conflated with other diseases such as leprosy. That said, artistic depictions of physical ailments will almost certainly prompt debate, while similarities among syndromes means that an examination of visual evidence will be confusing, perhaps even impossible, when attempting to differentiate between them.[1]

Nineteenth-century medical books will prove valuable in this endeavour, as they frequently include detailed illustrations meant to help physicians in diagnosis and treatment.

---

[1] Misidentification of a disease in an artwork carries the risk of impeding scholarly advances, as seen in the case of an illumination thought for many years to depict fourteenth-century plague victims that was instead an image of leprosy: see Green, Walker-Meikle, and Müller, "Diagnosis of a Plague Image." The possibility that some cases of leprosy may have been syphilis now means that the identification of all such images needs to be reevaluated.

The *Atlas Of Syphilis* (1898) by Franz Mraček, for example, is highly recommended for both its visual and written descriptions of the disease.[2] The photographs in Ernest Grin's study of endemic treponematosis in mid-twentieth-century Bosnia are also invaluable for learning about common symptoms.[3] Typical signs that historians will need to look for include, but are not restricted to: rashes, sores, and lesions on the skin, perhaps especially serpiginous phagedena; collapsed nasal bridge; Hutchinson's incisors and Moon's molars; swollen lips; protruding tongue; scars at the corners of the mouth; eighth nerve deafness; balding with cranial scarring; frontal bossing (protruding forehead); severe headaches, especially at night; bowed tibia; and the eye complaint interstitial keratitis, a symptom of congenital syphilis that causes chronic inflammation of the cornea leading to clouded vision and sometimes blindness.[4]

A manuscript illumination from the fourteenth-century encyclopedia, the *Omne Bonum*, may serve to illustrate the challenges of interpretation ahead for historians seeking to investigate possible representations of treponematosis in works of art. It shows a barber surgeon extracting a tooth from a patient with large pliers that have morphed into a snake with teeth protruding from its skin. The teeth have notches reminiscent of Hutchinson's incisors, as shown in a modern drawing of the deformity, although that is not definitive. More important is the fact that medieval contemporaries believed tooth pain—and sometimes headaches—to be

---

2 It is available from the Wellcome Institute Collection at https://wellcomecollection.org/works/nmjgtt7b.

3 Grin, "Endemic Syphilis in Bosnia" (1952). They remain under copyright and cannot be reproduced, but the article is open access on the World Health Organization website at https://www.who.int/publications/i/item/bulletin-1952-0701-1-74.

4 According to Cole and Jeans, interstitial keratitis is "the most frequently found lesion of late congenital syphilis": *Syphilis in Mother and Child* (1940), 16. See also Nabarro, *Congenital Syphilis* (1954), 329.

caused by a worm, as noted in the writings of the physician Gilbertus Anglicus (ca. 1180–ca. 1250).[5] It is more likely, however, that the illumination is a visual reference to "serpentine disease," an early name for syphilis that arose from a tendency of phagedenic lesions to spread on one side as they healed on the other, seeming to move like a serpent. Mraček describes the lesions this way: "If several nodes develop at once and undergo rapid disintegration, large sinuous ulcers appear. If the process continues and a new infiltrate is formed at the periphery, the ulcer becomes flattened on one side, but extends its limits on the other by fresh decay of the infiltrate, and we thus get serpiginous ulcers, semicircular or reniform [kidney-shaped] in shape, with scar formation at the center and ulceration at the freshly infiltrated periphery."[6] A better understanding of the relationship between syphilitic lesions and deformed teeth could also explain why people believed in the theory of tooth decay caused by worms.

According to Lucy Freeman Sandler, who has studied the *Omne Bonum* in detail, its compiler James le Palmer was very interested in the illustrations for his book, which were numerous. As she writes, "James [...] was especially receptive and sensitive to pictorial imagery as a carrier of meaning. He was, after all, an artist himself, expressing his own responses to the texts that he had compiled in figural as well as literal form through his elaborate graphic variations on the standard device of the scholarly commentator, the marginal manicule." The involvement of James in the book's program of illustration makes it more likely that he was responsible for including

---

5 Gerabek, "The Tooth-Worm" (1999); Getz, *Healing and Society*, 94–96.

6 See his *Atlas of Syphilis* (1898), 33. For an example of a serpiginous lesion see Grin, "Endemic Syphilis in Bosnia" (1952), fig. 18. The name "serpentine disease" may also have come from the meandering red rash that often appeared on the skin of the torso in syphilis, as illustrated in plate 15 of Mraček's study. Finally, and less literally, the name may be a reference to the devil, or serpent, who tempts Christians into committing sexual sins.

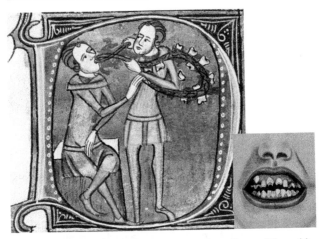

Figures 11 and 12. The illumination is from *Omne Bonum* (*Circumcisio–Dona Spiritui Sancti*). England, ca. 1360–1375. British Library, MS Royal 6 E VI, fol. 503v. © British Library Board. The watercolour drawing is from a nineteenth-century clinical study by Leonard Portal Mark, "Teeth from a Patient Affected by Inherited Syphilis. St Bartholomew's Hospital Archives & Museum." Wellcome Collection.

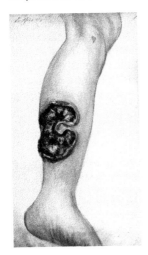

Figure 13. This diseased tissue on the calf of a woman's leg shows a serpiginous phagedena (ulcer). As Hutchinson describes the well-known "horseshoe sore" in his Syphilis: New and Enlarged Edition (1910), it was "a form of syphilitic lupoid affection of the skin, always tertiary, and always tending, unless stopped by treatment, to spread at its edge. To this quality of edge-spreading the term 'serpiginous' is applicable (p. 100)." Watercolour by C. D'Alton, 1857. Wellcome Collection.

the snake, which Sandler says differs from other illustrations in medieval medical books.[7] Significantly, given our discussion of the appearance of eels in St. Christopher stained-glass windows and wall paintings in England and Wales, W. E. Gerabek tells us that "In England [...] it was thought that the tooth-worm looked like an eel."[8]

The remaining images reproduced here were chosen to illustrate various common symptoms of treponematosis. In the condition called saddle nose, for instance, the spirochete invades the naso-palatal region, causing the bone to decay and collapse. It will probably be the easiest symptom for art historians to identify. Several examples are included here (Figures 14, 16, 17, 19–21, 23). Readers should also consult the work of Wieslaw Grzegorczyk, Joanna Grzegorczyk, and Krzysztof Grzegorczyk on the Veit Stoss Altarpiece in St. Mary's Church in Kraków. Although Stoss completed his work in 1489, it holds two clear examples of saddle nose deformity.[9]

For demonstrating the existence of syphilis in medieval times, it is significant that artists almost invariably included at least one man with a collapsed nasal bridge in scenes of the Passion. The deformity can be found among the men who arrest Christ, whip and ridicule him, and lead him to be crucified. In an era when people viewed physical deformity as evidence of sin, the association of saddle nose with men so evil they were willing to kill the son of God indicates it was the venereal form of the disease artists had in mind. This is useful evidence not only that artists recognized the presence of syphilis in the population, but also that they understood its relationship to the sin of sexual promiscuity. One illuminator went so far as to depict a flagellant with his penis exposed,

---

7 Sandler, *Omne Bonum*, 1:32, 1:91.

8 See Gerabek, "The Tooth-Worm" (1999), 2.

9 See their "Alleged Cases of Syphilis," where they note the earlier work of dermatologist and venereologist Franciszek Walter, "Wit Stwosz—rzeźbiarz chorób skórnych, szczegóły dermatologiczne Ołtarza Mariackiego" [Veit Stoss—The Sculptor of Skin Diseases, Dermatological Details of St. Mary's Altar in Krakow] (1933).

bright red at the tip, as though it were infected with a syphilitic chancre, which was probably the point (Figure 22).

Other images in this collection show a man ill with *syphilis papulosa* (Figure 25), a victim undergoing the sweating cure (Figure 27) and a man who has recovered from the worst effects of the disease but who shows its effects: scars at the corners of his mouth and a damaged left eye (Figure 29). Illuminations of individuals deemed to be insane reveal that a protruding tongue was regarded as a typical behaviour, probably resulting from treatment with mercury to induce salivation (Figures 23 and 24).[10] Illustrations of bowed tibia will prove more difficult to distinguish from other leg injuries, but along with depictions of headaches (Figure 31), hair loss (Figures 17, 21, and 23), and particular types of scarring that are common to many diseases, they can be employed effectively when used in conjunction with written or other visual sources.[11]

---

10 On mercury as a treatment for syphilis, see Arrizabalaga, Henderson, and French, *The Great Pox* (1997), 83–84, 139–44; Holcomb, "The Antiquity of Syphilis" (1935), 317–20.

11 Hair loss is discussed in detail in Berco, "The Great Pox" (2015), 232–36.

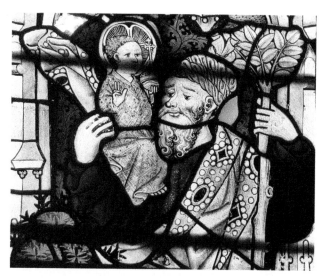

Figure 14. A stained-glass window from the fifteenth century depicts St. Christopher and the Christ child. The oddly shaped nose of the saint points to collapse of the nasal bridge resulting in saddle nose, a symptom of treponematosis. His small teeth also point to congenital syphilis, as observed by Hutchinson. The fact that the mouth was painted open to show the teeth makes it likely they were meant to convey some meaning, for medieval artists did not usually show teeth in their work as they were considered ugly. St Leonard Church. Bledington, Gloucestershire. © Jean McCreanor 2021

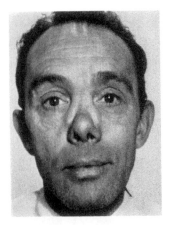

Figures 15 and 16. This photograph of an individual afflicted with saddle nose in modern times reveals a similar appearance to that of St. Christopher, with a depressed region where the bone has been lost on the bridge of the nose. It appears in McLaren and Penney, "The Reconstruction of the Syphilitic Saddle Nose" (1957–1958), figure 3. The gryllus with its remarkably similar facial configuration is from an early fourteenth-century book of hours, *The Maastricht Hours*, that includes several images of what appear to be saddle noses, including the ones below. Liège, Netherlands. © British Library Board, Stowe 17, fol. 151r.

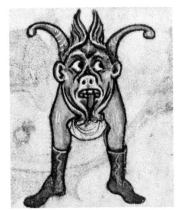

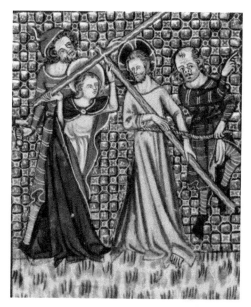

Figures 17. *The Taymouth Hours*, made in England in the second quarter of the fourteenth century, holds this image of Jesus carrying his cross to Golgotha. One of the men accompanying him has a nose with its tip pointing upward and prominent nostrils, perhaps a saddle nose. © British Library Board, Yates Thompson 13 fol. 120v.

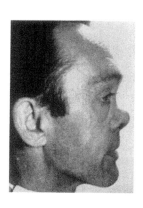

Figure 18. The modern photograph of a man at right shows the way a nose deformed by *Treponema pallidum* points upward. It appears in McLaren and Penney, "The Reconstruction of the Syphilitic Saddle Nose" (1957–1958), figure 3.

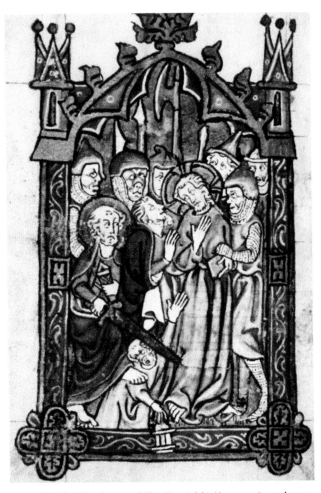

Figure 19. The illuminator of *The Maastricht Hours* portrayed some Roman soldiers with noses that have collapsed nasal bridges resembling saddle noses with their prominent, upturned nostrils. Here the servant of the Jewish high priest Caiaphas has the same deformity. Liège, Netherlands, first quarter of the fourteenth century. © British Library Board, Stowe 17, fol. 52v.

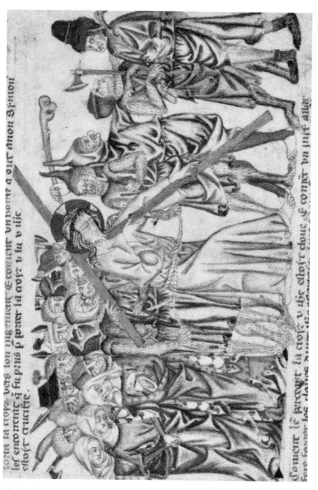

Figure 20. *The Holkham Bible Picture Book*, made in England ca. 1327-1335, has seven images showing Roman soldiers and citizens with saddle noses. This illumination shows three examples in one scene, indicating the artist's belief that the deformity was common at the time of the crucifixion. © British Library Board, Additional 47682, fol. 31.

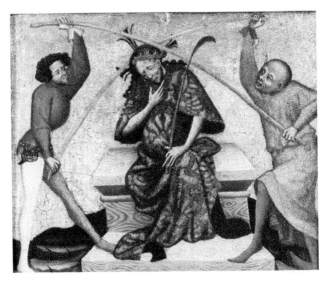

Figure 21. Here a healthy man and a man who is a victim of trepo-nematosis, probably syphilis, torment Christ before his crucifixion. The diseased man shows evidence of a collapsed nasal bridge and frontal bossing accompanied by baldness. His lips appear to be swollen, a condition Hutchinson observed in "constitutional" syphilis caused by chronic sores on the undersides of the lips: Syphilis (1910), Plate 13. Diptych with the Passion of Christ, ca. 1400 (detail). Austria, Styria. Cleveland Museum of Art.

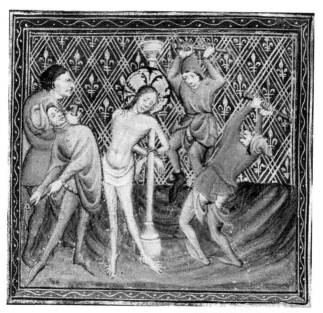

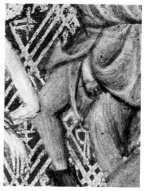

Figure 22. The man whose penis is exposed in this scene of the flagellation falls within the iconographical tradition of King David's fool. In the thirteenth and fourteenth centuries illuminators often painted him scantily clothed, without pants, or even naked. Significantly, Psalm 14 refers to a man who does not believe in God as a fool, a point relevant to the meaning of this illumination. Foolish men who did not believe in God were undoubtedly regarded as more likely to contract syphilis. From a French Book of Hours, ca. 1400–1410. J. Paul Getty Museum, MS Ludwig IX 4, fol. 47v.

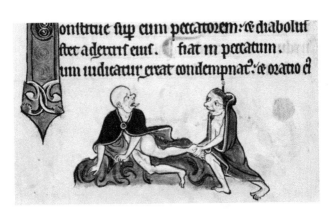

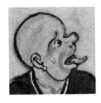

Figures 23 (with detail) and 24. A naked man showing signs of treponemal disease—collapsed nasal bridge, frontal bossing, and baldness—seems distressed as he lies on the ground near a companion who grasps his foot. His lined cape with brooch indicates he was once well-to-do. Perhaps he is suffering from a symptom of tertiary syphilis, general paresis, because his protruding tongue indicates insanity. We can see this from an entry in a medical book on the danger of being bitten by a madman, illustrated with a picture of a man sticking out his tongue. The author tells us that if the man were not mad but fasting, his bite was equally dangerous. This points to treatment with mercury accompanied by fasting, as was common later in cases of the French Pox. In either case it appears medical writers understood that the bite of some men could be deadly, which would certainly be true in cases of treponematosis whether they had progressed to general paresis or not. The illumination of the bald man comes from a thirteenth-century English psalter, *The Rutland Psalter*. © British Library Board, Additional 62925, fol. 110v. The image of the deranged man is from John Arderne's *Liber medicinarum*. England, first quarter of the fifteenth century. © British Library Board, Sloane 56, fol. 65.

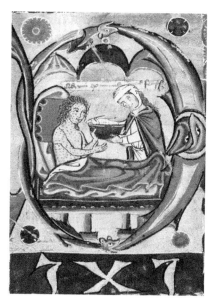

Figure 25. A man ill with a bad rash accepts a meal from a nun. The fact that she hands him a bowl with a large fish, as well as the decorative element of fish chosen by the artist for the initial letter "D" in which the scene appears, points to the nature of his disease—syphilis. Medieval viewers would have understood the fish symbolism and the moral lesson it conveyed. From a Swiss psalter, 1275-1300. J. Paul Getty Museum, MS Ludwig VIII 3, fol. 43.

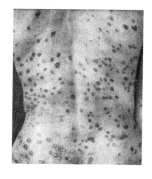

Figure 26. In untreated secondary syphilis, a rash usually covers the entire body. The papules can be either large or small, but they are generally the same size and brightly colored: "raw ham or coppery" as physician Selden I. Rainforth described them in the text accompanying the photograph shown here. Stereo photograph (detail), 1910. J. Paul Getty Museum, Object Number 84.XC.759.29.90.

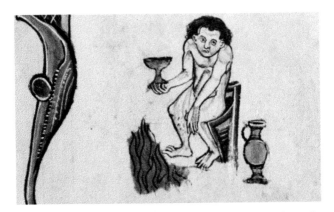

Figure 27. Treatment of syphilis often involved sweating in front of a fire to expel evil substances from the body brought on by humoral imbalance. Here, a man with spots on his leg sits in a fine chair and drinks from a golden cup, revealing he is a member of the elite. *The Rutland Psalter*, England, ca. 1260. © British Library Board, Additional 62925, fol. 109r.

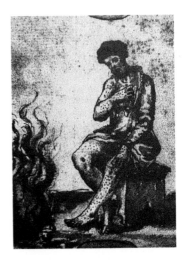

Figure 28. A patient with the French Pox sweats in front of a similar fire. This image from the sixteenth century helps us understand the meaning of the medieval Illumination. Italy. Biblioteca Comunale Augusta, Perugia, MS 472 (G61).

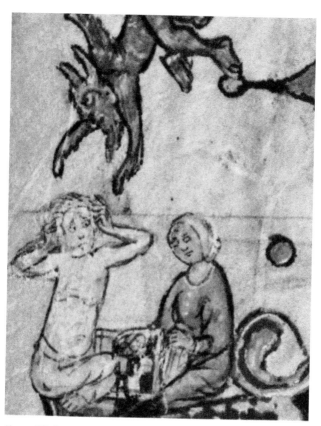

Figure 29. A man looks distressed and grimaces as if in pain as he holds his head with both hands. The devil flying toward him from above indicates that this is no ordinary head pain. Depictions of headaches in the absence of accompanying explanatory text will always be controversial, but this illumination appears in a manuscript that includes others depicting symptoms of treponemal disease. Multiple suggestive images in a manuscript can serve as an indication that the creators understood some aspects of the disease. *The Maastricht Hours*. Liège, Low Countries, first quarter of the fourteenth century. British Library, MS Stowe 17, fol. 111v (detail). © British Library Board.

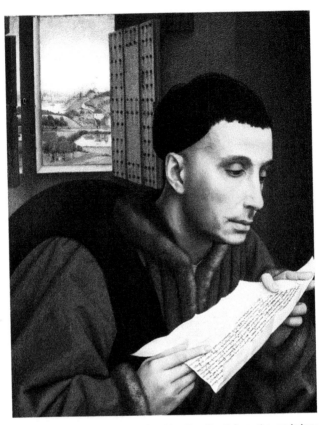

Figure 30. The elite subject of "A Man Reading," from the workshop of Rogier van der Weyden (ca. 1399–1464), has a scar at the corner of his mouth. Although it is impossible to know what caused the scar, the location and appearance indicate it could have resulted from a fissure commensurate with either congenital treponematosis or a case of acquired syphilis in adulthood. Oddly, the man is holding the letter to his right, yet his left eye is gazing in the opposite direction. The left eye is also painted a dull gray rather than brown like the right eye. All these clues point to interstitial keratitis, a symptom of congenital treponematosis, perhaps leading to blindness in the man's left eye.
© National Gallery, London / Art Resource, NY.

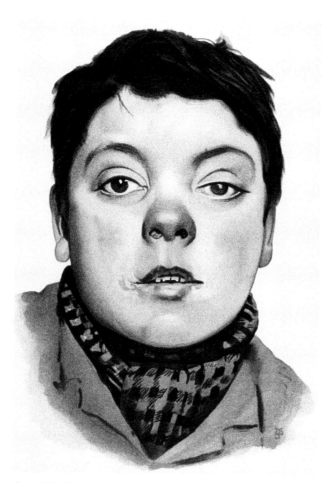

Figure 31. This chromolithograph of a young man with congenital syphilis depicts several symptoms of the disease. The victim has a dull left eye indicating interstitial keratitis accompanied by ptosis of the eyelid, a saddle nose with infectious debris in one nostril, Hutchinson's incisors, and fissures at the corners of his mouth due to rhagades. It was created for Byrom Bramwell's *Atlas of Clinical Medicine* (vol. 3, 1896). Science History Images / Alamy Stock Photo.

Conclusion

Paleopathologists have encountered difficulty in finding skeletal evidence of treponemal disease in premodern European cemeteries. Perhaps they would do better to study the remains of the royals and nobles housed in great cathedrals and abbeys. It seems possible that their luck will improve. If the remains of Edward IV could be examined, for example, they might reveal evidence of treatment with mercury. When used in doses that were too high or frequent, mercury was dangerous and could cause death. Among other conditions, it could provoke apoplexy.[1] It is entirely possible, then, that mercury poisoning contributed to the death of Edward IV by causing a stroke. His physicians and advisers would have understood this, which helps to explain why some people believed the king had been poisoned.

The skeleton of Henry VIII, who suffered at the end of his life from leg ulcers that may have caused painful periosteal infections or even necrosis of the leg bones themselves,

---

1 Holcomb, "The Antiquity of Syphilis" (1935), 318, citing Avicenna / Ibn Sina (980–1037), a polymath and philosopher who wrote the most highly regarded and influential medical treatise of the Middle Ages. Schwarz, Skytte, and Rasmussen tested the skeletons they studied for evidence of mercury. As they observe, "Mercury poisoning almost never leads to pathological bone lesions, but can be detected in bones as well as in teeth and hair samples by cold vapour atomic absorption spectroscopy." See their "Pre-Columbian Treponemal Infection in Denmark?" (2013), 4.

might also be instructive. Even more so might the remains of his children, eight of whom were stillborn or died in infancy. As Montiel and his co-authors have taught us, cases of congenital syphilis are most likely to bear the stigmata of the disease. In addition to these lost children, two of Henry's sons, Edward VI and the illegitimate Henry Fitzroy, duke of Richmond and Somerset, died in their teenage years, Edward supposedly of tuberculosis and Fitzroy of a pulmonary infection. We have good information about the condition of Edward's lungs because an autopsy was performed. According to the surgeon's report, "The disease whereof his majesty died was the disease of lungs, which had in them two great ulcers, and were putrefied." The previous year, Edward had suffered from a bad case of measles *and* smallpox, as he described his rash to a correspondent. His health never recovered. It certainly is possible, then, that he died of complications from congenital syphilis.[2] His half-brother Fitzroy may have done so as well, for pulmonary infections are completely consistent with the disease.[3] In any event, their cases are worth reconsidering, and perhaps their teeth and bones as well.

Barring permission to exhume the burials of royals and nobles, historians might want to reconsider the illnesses, patterns of child mortality, and causes of death of elites, and place them within an analytical framework that takes syphilis into account. It was noted long ago that noble families in medieval and early modern England had difficulty maintaining their family lines due to the absence of male heirs.[4] Perhaps Henry VIII was not the only magnate to have his dynastic plans ruined by the venereal form of treponematosis, a *mort male* indeed.

---

2 Beverley Murphy, "Fitzroy, Henry," and Dale Hoak, "Edward VI," in the *Oxford Dictionary of National Biography*.

3 Futami et al., "A Lung Abscess Caused by Secondary Syphilis" (2019), 598; Florencio et al., "Secondary Syphilis with Pulmonary Involvement Mimicking Lymphoma" (2019); and Azusu et al., "Secondary Syphilis with Pulmonary Involvement" (2018).

4 Stone, *The Crisis of the Aristocracy*, 169.

Bibliography

Akwari, F. "Is Bejel Syphilis?" *British Journal of Venereal Diseases* 25 (1949): 115–23.

Álvarez, Alicia Rodriguez, and M. Victoria Dominguez Rodriguez. "Moral Considerations on Female Sexuality in Late Medieval English Scientific Treatises." In *Voices on the Past: Studies in Old and Middle English Language and Literature*, edited by Alicia Rodriguez Álvarez and Francisco Alonso Almeida, 49–62. A Coruña: Netbiblo, 2004.

Arrizabalaga, Jon. "The Changing Identity of the French Pox in Early Renaissance Castile." In *Between Text and Patient: The Medical Enterprise in Medieval and Early Modern Europe*, edited by Florence Eliza Glaze and Brian K. Nance, 397–417. Florence: SISMEL, 2011.

Arrizabalaga, Jon, John Henderson, and Roger French. *The Great Pox: The French Disease in Renaissance Europe*. New Haven: Yale University Press, 1997.

Azusu, Ohta et al. "Secondary Syphilis with Pulmonary Involvement." *Internal Medicine* 57 (2018): 121–26.

Baker, Brenda J. et al. "Advancing the Understanding of Treponemal Disease in the Past and Present." *Yearbook of Physical Anthropology* 171 (2020): 5–41.

Baker, Brenda J., and George Armelagos. "The Origin and Antiquity of Syphilis: Paleopathological Diagnosis and Interpretation." *Current Anthropology* 29 (1988): 703–37.

Bari, Arfan Ul. "Early Syphilis Presenting as Anal Fissure: A Case Report." *Journal of Pakistan Association of Dermatologists* 15 (2005): 92–95.

Basin, Thomas. *Histoire des règnes de Charles VII et de Louis XI*. Edited by Jules Étienne Joseph Quicherat. 4 vols. Paris: Renouard, 1855–59.

[Batman, Stephen]. *Batman vppon Bartholome his Booke De Proprietatibus Rerum, Newly Corrected, Enlarged and Amended*. London: Thomas East, 1582.

Bennett, Judith M. "Death and the Maiden." *Journal of Medieval and Early Modern Studies* 42 (2012): 269–305.

Berco, Cristian. "The Great Pox, Symptoms, and Social Bodies in Early Modern Spain." *Social History of Medicine* 28 (2015): 225–44.

Betcher, Gloria J. "A Tempting Theory: What Early Cornish Mermaid Images Reveal About the First Doctor's Analogy in *Passio Domini*." *The Early Drama, Art, and Music Review* 18 (1996): 65–76.

Bible Moralisée: Codex Vindobonensis 2554, Vienna, Österreichischen Nationalbibliothek. Translated with commentary by Gerald B. Guest. London: Harvey Miller, 1995.

Blondiaux, Joël. "La Paléopathologie des tréponématoses." In *Ostéo-archéologie et techniques médico-légales: Tendances et perspectives. Pour un manuel pratique de paléopathologie humaine*, edited by Philippe Charlier, 453–62. Paris: De Boccard, 2008.

Boehrer, Bruce Thomas. "Early Modern Syphilis." *Journal of the History of Sexuality* 1 (1990): 197–214.

Bouwman, Abigail, and Terence A. Brown. "The Limits of Bio-molecular Palaeopathology: Ancient DNA Cannot Be Used to Study Venereal Syphilis." *Journal of Archaeological Science* 32 (2005): 703–13.

Brundage, James. "Concubinage and Marriage in Medieval Canon Law." *Journal of Medieval History* 1 (1975): 1–17.

Calendar of State Papers and Manuscripts Existing in the Archives and Collections of Milan. Vol. 1 (1385–1618). Edited by Allen B. Hinds. London: His Majesty's Stationery Office, 1912.

Camille, Michael. "Manuscript Illumination and the Art of Copulation." In *Constructing Medieval Sexuality*, edited by Karma Lochrie, Peggy McCracke, and James A. Schultz, 58–90. Minneapolis: University of Minnesota Press, 1997.

Citrome, Jeremy J. *The Surgeon in Medieval English Literature.* New York: Palgrave Macmillan, 2006.

Cole, Garrard, and Tony Waldron. "Apple Down 152: A Putative Case of Syphilis from Sixth Century AD Anglo-Saxon England." *American Journal of Physical Anthropology* 144 (2011): 72–79.

——. "Letter to the Editor: Apple Down 152 Putative Syphilis: Pre-Colombian Date Confirmed." *American Journal of Physical Anthropology* 156 (2014): 489.

——. "Letter to the Editor: Syphilis Revisited." *American Journal of Physical Anthropology* 149 (2012): 149–50.

Cole, Harold N., and Philip C. Jeans. *Syphilis in Mother and Child.* Printed for the Federal Security Agency. Washington, DC: United States Government Printing Office, 1940.

Commines, Philippe de de. *Memoirs.* Translated by Isabelle Cazeaux and edited by Samuel Kinser. 2 vols. Columbia: University of South Carolina Press, 1969.

Cox, Daniel R. A. et al. "Syphilis as an Atypical Cause of Peri-anal Fissure." *Journal of Surgical Case Reports* for 2018, no. 11 (2018): rjy320. doi:10.1093/jscr/rjy320.

The Crowland Chronicle Continuations: 1459–1486. Edited and translated by Nicholas Pronay and John Cox. London: Richard III and Yorkist History Trust, 1986.

Davies, John David Griffith. *Henry V.* London: Barker, 1935.

Erasmus, Desiderius. *Adages III iv 1 to IV ii 100.* Translated and annotated by Denis L. Drysdall. Edited by John N. Grant. Collected Works of Erasmus 35. Toronto: University of Toronto Press, 2005.

Erdal, Yilmaz Selim. "A Pre-Columbian Case of Congenital Syphilis from Anatolia (Nicaea, 13th Century AD)." *International Journal of Osteoarchaeology* 16 (2006): 16–33.

Fabricius, Johannes. *Syphilis in Shakespeare's England.* London Kingsley, 1994.

Florencio, Kelwya Bruna Vasconcelos et al. "Secondary Syphilis with Pulmonary Involvement Mimicking Lymphoma: A Case Report." *Revista da Sociedade Brasileira de Medicina Tropical* 52 (2019): https://doi.org/10.1590/0037-8682-0044-2019.

Fraser, Claire M. et al. "Complete Genome Sequence of *Treponema pallidum*, the Syphilis Spirochete." *Science* 281 (1998): 375–88.

Futami, Shinji et al. "A Lung Abscess Caused by Secondary Syphilis—The Utility of Polymerase Chain Reaction Techniques in Transbronchial Biopsy: A Case Report." *BMC Infectious Diseases* 19, no. 598 (2019): https://doi.org/10.1186/s12879-019-4236-4.

Gascoigne, Thomas. *Loci e libro veritatum: Passages Selected from Gascoigne's Theological Dictionary Illustrating the Condition of Church and State, 1403–1458.* With an introduction by James E. Thorold Rogers. Oxford: Clarendon, 1881.

Gaul, Johanna Sophia et al. "A Probable Case of Congenital Syphilis from Pre-Columbian Austria." *Anthropologischer Anzeiger* 72 (2015): 451–72.

Gerabek, Werner E. "The Tooth-Worm: Historical Aspects of a Popular Medical Belief." *Clinical Oral Investigations* 3 (1999): 1–6.

Getz, Faye M. *Healing and Society in Medieval England: A Middle English Translation of the Pharmaceutical Writings of Gilbertus Anglicus*. Madison: University of Wisconsin Press, 1991.

Giancarni, Lorenzo, and Sheila A. Lukehart, "The Endemic Treponematoses." *Clinical Microbiology Reviews* 27 (2014): 89–115.

Giffin, Karen et al. "A Treponemal Genome from an Historic Plague Victim Supports a Recent Emergence of Yaws and its Presence in 15th Century Europe." *Scientific Reports* 10, no. 9499 (2020): https://doi.org/10.1038/s41598-020-66012-x.

Gładykowska-Rzeczycka, Judyta, et al. "Treponematosis in a 14th-Century Skeleton from Wroclaw, Poland." *Journal of Paleopathology* 15 (2003): 187–97.

Goens, Julien L., Camila K. Janniger, and K. De Wolf. "Dermatologic and Systemic Manifestations of Syphilis." *American Family Physician* 50 (1994): 1013–21.

Green, Monica H. "The Four Black Deaths." *The American Historical Review* 125 (2020): 1601–31.

——. ed. *Pandemic Disease in the Medieval World: Rethinking the Black Death*. Leeds: Arc Humanities, 2015. Also published as the inaugural issue of *The Medieval Globe* 1 (2014).

Green, Monica H., Kathleen Walker-Meikle, and Wolfgang P. Müller. "Diagnosis of a Plague Image: A Cautionary Tale." In *Pandemic Disease in the Medieval World: Rethinking the Black Death*, edited by Monica H. Green, 309–22. Leeds: Arc Humanities, 2015.

Grin, Ernest I. "Endemic Syphilis in Bosnia: Clinical and Epidemiological Observations on a Successful Mass-Treatment Campaign." *Bulletin of the World Health Organization* 7 (1952): 1–74.

Grzegorczyk, Wieslaw, Joanna Grzegorczyk, and Krzysztof Grzegorczyk. "Alleged Cases of Syphilis Immortalized in the Krakow Altarpiece by Veit Stoss in the Light of New Research on the Origins of the Disease in Europe." *Medical Review* 14 (2016): 340–57.

Guerra, Francisco. "The Dispute over Syphilis: Europe versus America." *Clio Medica: Acta Academiae Internationalis Historiae Medicinae* 13 (1978): 39–61.

——. "The European-American Exchange." *History and Philosophy of the Life Sciences* 15 (1993): 313–27.

Hackett, Cecil J. *Diagnostic Criteria of Syphilis, Yaws, and Treponarid (Treponematoses) and of some Other Diseases in Dry Bones.* Berlin: Springer, 1976.

——. "The Human Treponematoses." In *Diseases in Antiquity: A Survey of the Diseases, Injuries, and Surgery of Early Populations*, edited by Don Brothwell and Andrew T. Sandison, 152–69. Springfield: Thomas, 1967.

Hanham, Alison. "The Mysterious Affair at Crowland Abbey." *The Ricardian* 18 (2008): 1–11.

Hardyng, John. *The Chronicle of John Hardyng, [...] together with the Continuation of Richard Grafton.* Edited by Henry Ellis. London: Rivington et al., 1812.

Harper, Kristin N. et al. "The Origin and Antiquity of Syphilis Revisited: An Appraisal of Old World Pre-Columbian Evidence for Treponemal Infection." *Yearbook of Physical Anthropology* 54 (2011): 99–133.

Henneberg, Maciej, and Renata J. Henneberg. "Treponematosis in an Ancient Greek Colony of Metaponto, Southern Italy,

580–250 BCE." In *L'Origine de la syphilis en Europe: avant ou après 1493?*, edited by Olivier Dutour et al., 92–98. Paris: Errance, 1994.

Hernando Garrido, José Luis. "San Cristóbal y la Sirenita: Aviso para Peregrinos y Navegantes / St. Christopher and the Little Mermaid: Warning for Pilgrims and Sailors." *Codex Aquilarensis* 29 (2013): 251–70.

Hicks, Michael. "The Second Anonymous Continuation of the Crowland Abbey Chronicle 1459–86 Revisited." *English Historical Review* 122 (2007): 349–70.

Hillson, Simon. *Dental Anthropology.* New York: Cambridge University Press, 1996.

Holcomb, Richmond C. "The Antiquity of Syphilis." *Medical Life* 42 (1935): 275–325.

——— . "Christopher Columbus and the American Origin of Syphilis." *United States Naval Medical Bulletin* 32 (1934): 1–30.

Hollings, R. M. "Syphilitic Ulcers of the Anus." *Proceedings of the Royal Society of Medicine* 54 (1961): 730–31.

Hudson, Ellis Herndon. "Historical Approach to the Terminology of Syphilis." *Archives of Dermatology* 84 (1961): 545–62.

——— . *Non-Venereal Syphilis: A Sociological and Medical Study of Bejel.* Edinburgh: Livingstone, 1958.

——— . "The Treponematoses—or Treponematosis?" *The British Journal of Venereal Diseases* 34 (1958): 22–23.

——— . "Treponematosis and Man's Social Evolution." *American Anthropologist* 67 (1965): 885–901.

——— . "A Unitarian View of Treponematosis." *American Journal of Tropical Medicine and Hygiene* 26 (1946): 135–39.

Hunnius, Tanya E. von et al. "Digging Deeper into the Limits of Ancient DNA Research on Syphilis." *Journal of Archaeological Science* 34 (2007): 2091–2100.

Hutchinson, Jonathan. *Syphilis*. New ed. New York: Funk and Wagnalls, 1910.

Ioannou, Stella, Renata J. Henneberg, and Maciej Henneberg. "Presence of Dental Signs of Congenital Syphilis in Pre-Modern Specimens." *Archives of Oral Biology* 85 (2018): 192–200.

Ioannou, Stella, Sadaf Sassani, Maciej Henneberg, and Renata J. Henneberg. "Diagnosing Congenital Syphilis Using Hutchinson's Method: Differentiating Between Syphilitic, Mercurial, and Syphilitic-Mercurial Dental Defects." *American Journal of Physical Anthropology* 159 (2016): 617–29.

Jacobus de Voragine. *The Golden Legend: or, Lives of the Saints, as Englished by William Caxton [1470]*. London: Dent, 1900.

——. *The Golden Legend: Readings on the Saints by Jacobus de Voragine*. Translated by William Granger Ryan with an introduction by Eamon Duffy. Princeton: Princeton University Press, 2012.

Jankauskas, Rimantas. "Syphilis in Eastern Europe: Historical and Paleopathological Evidence." In *L'Origine de la syphilis en Europe: avant ou après 1493?*, edited by Olivier Dutour et al., 237–39. Paris: Errance, 1994.

Jones, Peter Murray. "Four Middle English Translations of John of Arderne." In *Latin and Vernacular: Studies in Late-Medieval Texts and Manuscripts*, 61–89, edited by A. J. Minnis. Cambridge: Brewer, 1989.

——. "John of Arderne and the Mediterranean Tradition of Scholastic Surgery." In *Practical Medicine from Salerno to the Black Death*, 289–321, edited by Luis García-Ballester et al., 289–321. Cambridge: Cambridge University Press, 1994.

——. "Staying with the Program: Illustrated Manuscripts of John of Arderne." *English Manuscript Studies, 1100-1700* 10 (2002): 204-27.

Jongh, Eddy de. "The Symbolism of Fish, Fisherman, Fishing Gear and the Catch." In *Fish: Still Lifes by Dutch and Flemish Masters*, edited by Liesbeth Helmus, 75-120. Utrecht: Centraal Museum, 2004.

The Julius Exclusus. Translated by Paul Pascal, with an introduction and critical notes by J. Kelly Sowards. Bloomington: Indiana University Press, 1968.

Kaplan, Gregory B. "The (Columbian) Myth of Syphilis: A Textual Perspective." *Hispanófila* 134 (2002): 21-35.

Kolman, Connie J. et al. "Identification of *Treponema Pallidum* Subspecies *Pallidum* in a 200-Year-Old Skeletal Specimen." *The Journal of Infectious Diseases* 180 (1999): 2060-63.

Letters and Papers, Foreign and Domestic of the Reign of Henry VIII, Preserved in the Public Record Office, the British Museum, and Elsewhere in England. Edited by James Gairdner *et al.* 21 vols. in 33 parts. London: Longman, Green, Longman, and Roberts [and other presses], 1862-1932.

Lelong, Olivia, and Julie A. Roberts. "St. Trolla's Chapel, Kintradwell, Sutherland: The Occupants of the Medieval Burial Ground and their Patron Saint." *Scottish Archaeological Journal* 25 (2003): 147-63.

McLaren, Lyall R., and Dennis Penney. "The Reconstruction of the Syphilitic Saddle Nose: A Review of Seven Cases." *British Journal of Plastic Surgery* 10 (1957-1958): 236-52.

McNiven, Peter. "The Problem of Henry IV's Health, 1405-1413." *English Historical Review* 100 (1985): 747-72.

Majander, Kerttu et al. "Ancient Bacterial Genomes Reveal a High Diversity of Treponema pallidum Strains in Early Modern Europe." *Current Biology* 30 (2020): 3788-3803.

Mancini, Domenico. *De occupatione regni Anglie per Reccardum tercium*. Translated as *The Usurpation of Richard III* by Charles A. Armstrong. 2nd ed. Oxford: Clarendon, 1969.

[Mandeville, John.] *The Defective Version of Mandeville's Travels*. Edited by M. C. Seymour. Early English Text Society, o.s., 319. Oxford: Oxford University Press, 2002.

Major, Ralph H. *Classic Descriptions of Disease: With Biographical Sketches of the Authors*. 3rd ed. Springfield: Thomas, 1945.

Mark, Leonard. "Teeth from a Patient Affected by Inherited Syphilis. St Bartholomew's Hospital Archives & Museum." wellcomecollection.org/works/fdfqb8ct.

Mays, Simon, Gillian Crane-Kramer, and Alex Bayliss. "Two Probable Cases of Treponemal Disease of Medieval Date from England." *American Journal of Physical Anthropology* 120 (2003): 133–43.

Mays, Simon, Stefanie Vincent, and J. Meadows. "A Possible Case of Treponemal Disease from England Dating to the 11th–12th Century AD." *International Journal of Osteoarchaeology* 22 (2012): 366–72.

Montiel, Rafael et al. "Neonate Human Remains: A Window of Opportunity to the Molecular Study of Ancient Syphilis." *PLoS ONE* 7, no. 5 (2012): e36371. https://doi.org/10.1371/journal.pone.0036371.

More, Thomas. *The History of King Richard III*. Edited by George M. Logan. Bloomington: Indiana University Press, 2005.

Mraček, Franz. *Atlas of Syphilis and the Venereal Diseases, Including a Brief Treatise on the Pathology and Treatment*. Authorized translation from the German. Edited by L. Bolton Bangs. Philadelphia: Saunders, 1898.

Nabarro, David. *Congenital Syphilis*. London: Arnold, 1954.

Ortner, Donald J. *Identification of Pathological Conditions in Human Skeletal Remains*. 2nd ed. San Diego: Academic, 2003.

Osler, William. *Aequanimitas: With Other Addresses to Medical Students, Nurses, and Practitioners of Medicine*. 2nd ed. Philadelphia: Blakiston's, 1910.

Oxford Dictionary of National Biography (online edition). Oxford: Oxford University Press, 2004–2021.

Payer, Pierre J. *The Bridling of Desire: Views of Sex in the Later Middle Ages*. Toronto: University of Toronto Press, 1993.

Power, D'Arcy. "The Lesser Writings of John Arderne." Seventeenth International Congress of Medicine, London, 1913 [1914], 107–33. https://wellcomecollection.org/works/j72nbhwq/items?canvas=3.

Pridgeon, Eleanor E. "Saint Christopher Wall Paintings in English and Welsh Churches c. 1250–c. 1500." PhD diss., University of Leicester, 2008.

Putoken, Tauno. "Dental Changes in Congenital Syphilis: Relationship to Other Syphilitic Stigmata." *Acta Dermato-Venereologica* 42 (1962): 44–62.

Quétel, Claude. *History of Syphilis*. Translated by Judith Braddock and Brian Pike. Baltimore: The Johns Hopkins University Press, 1990.

Roberts, Charlotte. "Treponematosis in Gloucester, England: A Theoretical and Practical Approach to the Pre-Columbian Theory." In *L'Origine de la syphilis en Europe, avant ou après 1493?*, edited by Olivier Dutour et al., 101–8. Paris: Errance, 1994.

Roberts, Charlotte, and Rebecca Redfern. "Bioarchaeological Contributions to Understanding the History of Treponemal Disease." In *The Hidden Affliction: Sexually Transmitted Infections and Infertility in History*, edited by Simon Szreter, 93–123. Rochester: Rochester University Press, 2019.

Rohan Book of Hours. With an introduction by Millard Meiss and an introduction and commentaries by Marcel Thomas. London: Thames and Hudson, 1973.

Román, Gustavo C., and Lydia N. Román. "Occurrence of Congenital, Cardiovascular, Visceral, Neurologic, and Neuro-Ophthalmologic Complications in Late Yaws: A Theme for Future Research." *Reviews of Infectious Diseases* 8 (1986): 760–70.

Ross, Charles. *Edward IV.* New Haven: Yale University Press, 1974.

Roye, Jean de. *Journal de Jean de Roye: Connu sous le nom de Chronique scandaleuse, 1460–1483.* Edited by Bernard de Mandrot. 2 vols. Paris: Renouard, 1894.

Rushforth, Gordon McNeil. *Medieval Christian Imagery: As Illustrated by the Painted Windows of Great Malvern Priory Church, Worcestershire.* Oxford: Clarendon, 1936.

Sandler, Lucy Freeman. *Omne Bonum: A Fourteenth-Century Encyclopedia of Universal Knowledge.* 2 vols. London: Harvey Miller, 1996.

Schuenemann, Verena J. et al. "Historic *Treponema pallidum* Genomes from Colonial Mexico Retrieved from Archaeological Remains." *PLoS Neglected Tropical Diseases* 12, no. 6 (2018): e0006447. https://doi.org/10.1371/journal.pntd.0006447.

Schwarz, Susanne, Lilian Skytte, and Kaare Lund Rasmussen. "Pre-Columbian Treponemal Infection in Denmark?—A Paleopathological and Archaeometric Approach." *Heritage Science* 1 (2013): 19.

Scofield, Cora L. *Life and Reign of Edward IV, King of England and France and Lord of Ireland.* 2 vols. New York: Longman, Green, 1923.

Steinbock, R. Ted. *Paleopathological Diagnosis and Interpretation.* Springfield: Thomas, 1976.

Stirland, Ann. *Criminals and Paupers: The Graveyard of St Margaret Fyebriggate in combusto, Norwich.* With contributions from Brian Ayers and Jayne Brown. East Anglian Archaeology

129. Dereham: Historic Environment, Norfolk Museums and Archaeology Service: 2009.

———. "Evidence for Pre-Columbian Treponematosis in Mediaeval Europe." In *L'Origine de la syphilis en Europe, avant ou après 1493?*, edited by Olivier Dutour et al., 109-15. Paris: Errance, 1994.

Stone, Anne C., and Andrew T. Ozga. "Ancient DNA in the Study of Ancient Disease." In *Ortner's Identification of Pathological Conditions in Human Skeletal Remains*, edited by Jane E. Buikstra, 183-210. 3rd ed. San Diego: Academic, 2019.

Stone, Lawrence. *The Crisis of the Aristocracy: 1558-1641*. Oxford: Clarendon, 1965.

Tampa, Mircea et al. "Brief History of Syphilis." *Journal of Medicine and Life* 7 (2014): 4-10.

Turner, Marion. "Illness Narratives in the Later Middle Ages: Arderne, Chaucer, and Hoccleve." *Journal of Medieval and Early Modern Studies* 46 (2016): 61-87.

———. "Thomas Usk and John Arderne." *The Chaucer Review* 47 (2012): 95-105.

Vergil, Polydore. *Three Books of Polydore Vergil's English History, Comprising the Reigns of Henry VI, Edward IV, and Richard III*. Edited by Henry Ellis. London: The Camden Society, 1844.

Walker, Don et al. "Evidence of Skeletal Treponematosis from the Medieval Burial Ground of St Mary Spital, London, and Implications for the Origins of the Disease in Europe." *American Journal of Physical Anthropology* 156 (2015): 90-101.

Weisenberg, Elliott. "Syphilis." *PathologyOutlines.com*, 2020. https://www.pathologyoutlines.com/topic/colonsyphilis.html.

Wroe, Ann. *The Perfect Prince: The Mystery of Perkin Warbeck and his Quest for the Throne of England*. New York: Random House, 2003.

Printed and bound by CPI Group (UK) Ltd, Croydon, CR0 4YY

12/06/2024

14514476-0002